BENCH PRESS
THE SCIENCE

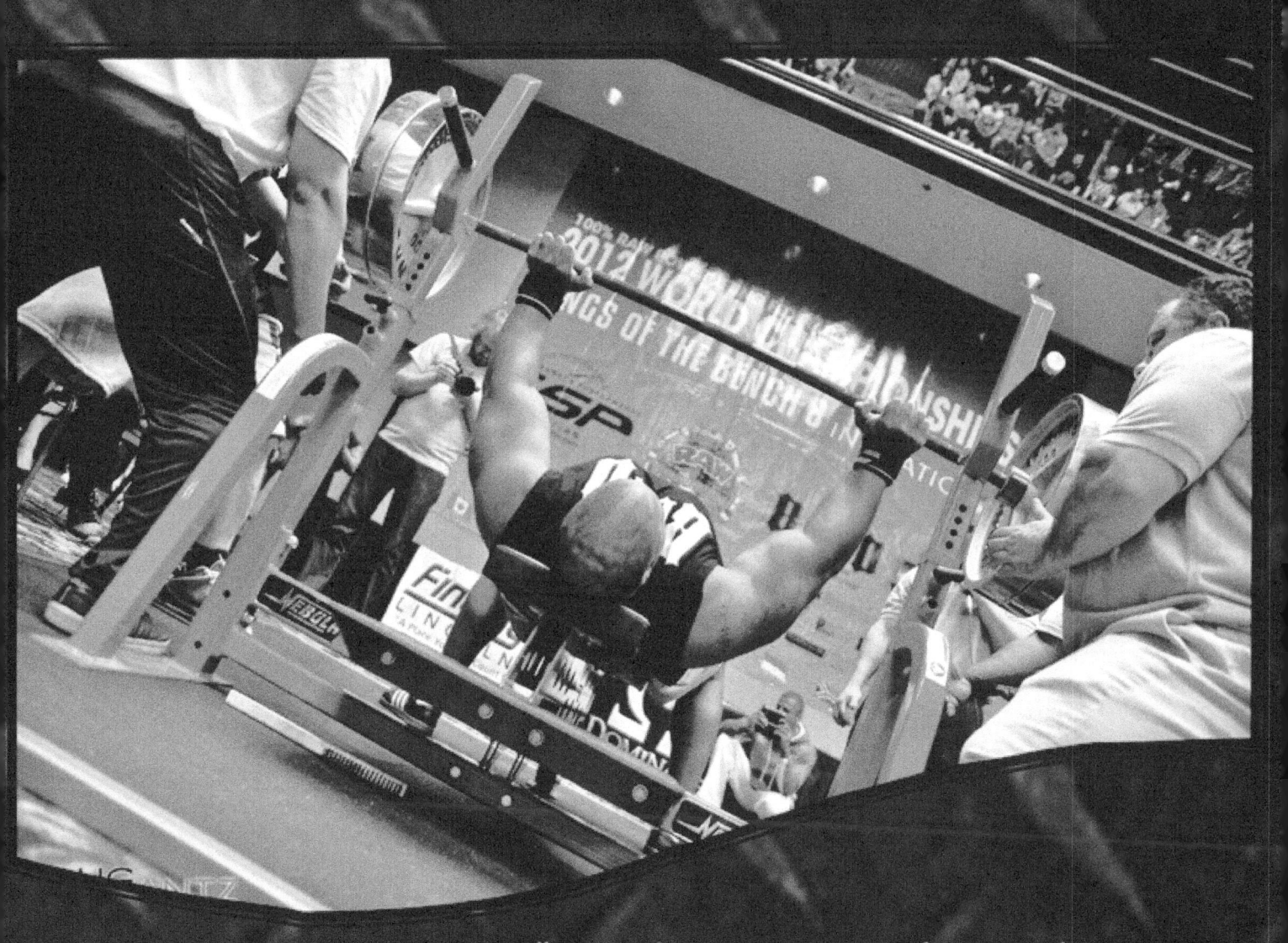

"....the most comprehensive book ever written on the bench press."

Eddy Coan

BY JOSH BRYANT
Author of Metroflex Gym Powerbuilding Basics

BENCH PRESS:

THE SCIENCE

BY JOSH BRYANT

Copyright © 2013 JoshStrength, LLC

All rights reserved, including file sharing, the right to reproduce this work, in whole or in part, in any form.

Dedication Page

. This book is dedicated to the memory of my friend, Ross Shreves. Ross was a great help in the editorial process of this book and a writing mentor for me. Ross had a 540-pound competition bench press and one of the best hearts of any person I have ever known. Ross's death cut short the career of a great teacher, friend and powerlifter. Ross is now in heaven with his Lord and Savior, Jesus Christ. I miss you brother and I am a better person for knowing you. There are pictures of Ross throughout the book.

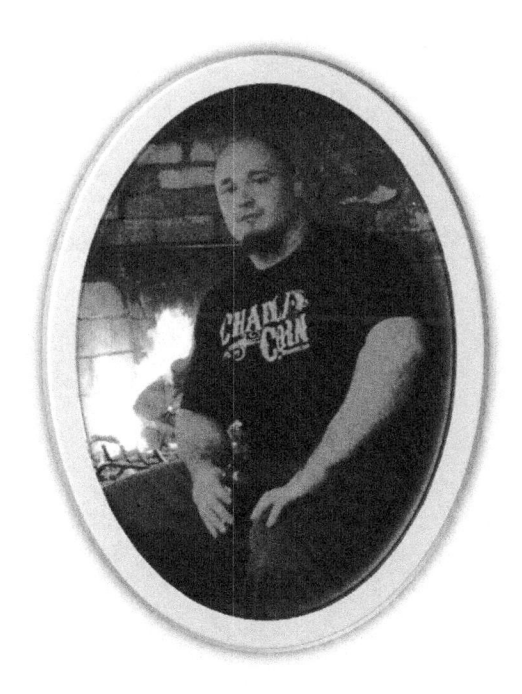

.

Picture Acknowledgements

I would like to thank the following people for providing illustrations

- Seanzilla Katterle of HardcorePowerlifting.com

- Dave Tate and Steve Colescott of Elitefts.com

- Legendary Muscle Sport Photographer Doug Jantz - www.dougjantzphotography.com

- Josh Windsor of Josh Windsor Photo and Design - HardcorePowerlifting.com

  Photographer

- Eric Spoto

- Michael Zundelevich

- Mark Bell creator of the Sling Shot of MarkBellPower.com

Contents

About the Author 8
The Bench Press 9
    Five "Bench Big" Strategies 10
    Raw and Equipped Bench Pressing 12
    Progression of the Bench Press World Record 13
    Progression of the Raw Bench Press World Record 14
    Progression of records 15
    Pandora's Box Opened 15
    Raw Bench Pressers Physiques 15
    Final Thoughts 17
Compensatory Acceleration Training (CAT) 18
    Lifting Heavy Weights Slowly? 19
    Field Test 19
    Kaz Sheds Light 20
    CAT Practically Applied 20
    Learning to Explode 21
    Muscle/Movement Intention Contrasted 22
    Any Lift Can Be Explosive 22
    CAT Efficiency 23
    Further CAT Benefits 24
    CAT Guidelines 25
    Speed - the Name of the Game 26
    Practical Application 27
    The Race is on with the Sticking Point 28
    Practical Application 29
    Compensatory Acceleration Training (CAT) Reigns Supreme 30
    Practical Application 31
    Practical Application 32
    CAT Training Continually Reigns Supreme 33
    Practical Application 33

  Tempo and Power Output 34

  Practical Application 34

  Final Thoughts 34

Elimination of Sticking Points: A Scientific Approach **35**

  What is an Isometric Contraction? 36

  Your CNS: The Predator, Not the Prey 37

  Determining Sticking Points 37

  Isometrics for the Bench Press 38

  Potential Causes of Sticking Points 38

  Speed and Sticking Points 38

  Isometrics and the PAP Effect 39

  Understanding Isometrics 39

  Isometrics, World Records and Pink Pills 40

  Isometric Drawbacks 43

  Training Benefits & Guidelines 44

  Quasi Isometrics 47

  The Risk to Benefit Ratio of Bench Press Specific Isometrics 48

  Functional Isometrics 49

  Functional Isometric Routine 50

  Isodynamics 51

  Isodynamic Routine 53

  Prison Yard Push Isometrics 54

  Isometric/CAT Contrast 55

  Isometric/CAT Contrast Routine 57

  Isometric Programming 58

  Sticking Points-Cause and Effect 59

  Practical Application 60

  Final Thoughts 60

The Power of Positive Benching **61**

  Dead Bench Practically Applied 61

  Positive Verses Negatives for Strength Gains 65

  Practical Applications 66

  Final Thoughts 67

Explosive Bench Pressing: Plyometrics and Throws 68
- Bench Press: Phase 1, 2, & 3 69
- Bench Press and Sprinting 69
- Turning Off Inhibitory Mechanisms 69
- Bench Press Specific Plyometrics 70
- Explosive Movements Activate Limit Strength in the Bench Press 72
- Practical Application 74
- Weight Releasers Increase Power 75
- Practical Application 75
- Wearing Off of Stretch Reflex Causes Sticking Point 76
- Practical Application 77
- Final Thoughts 77

Sound Science or Bro Science? 78
- Muscle Activation: Fat Bar verses Standard Bar 79
- Practical Application 79
- Static Stretching and the Bench Press 79
- Practical Application 80
- Final Thoughts 80

Partials for Raw Bench Pressers 81
- Board Presses 81
- 12 Week Full ROM Injury: Board Press Cycle 82
- Board Press Transference 82
- Progressive Distance Training 83
- Rack lockout overloads 84
- Partial Overload Training 85
- Practical Application 85
- Final Thoughts 86

Bands and Chains for the Raw Bench Presser 87
- Bands Enhance Bench Press Strength and Power 88
- Practical Applications 88
- Train with Chains and Bench More 89
- Practical Application 89
- Bench Press with Chains: Strength Gains, Shoulder Pain and Muscle Soreness 90

- Practical Application 91
- Bar Speed: Barbell Verses Barbell with Chains 93
- Practical Application: 94
- Final Thoughts 94

Bench Press: Muscle Activation, Technique, and Volume 96
- Grip Width-Shoulder Safety and Muscle Activation 96
- Practical Application 97
- Factoring in Rest Intervals in Program Design 97
- Practical Application 98
- Failure Affects Bar Path 99
- Practical Application 100
- Big Al Davis' Bench Press Workout 101
- Big Al Davis' Rest-Pause Grinding Strength Workout 101
- Dumbbells, Free Weight, Machines: the Differences 102
- Practical Application 102
- Practice How You Play 103
- Practical Application 104
- Technical Differences: Elite and Novice Bench Press 104
- Practical Application 105
- How Many Sets? 105
- Practical Application 105
- Another Case for Volume 105
- Practical Application 106
- Final Thoughts 106

Science and the Sling Shot 107
- Final Thoughts 109

Miscellaneous Bench Press Science 110
- Curls Are For Girls and So Are Bench Presses 110
- Practical Application 111
- Take Caffeine and Bench Press More 111
- Practical Application: 112
- Complex Training Saves Time 112
- Practical Application 112

- Restricting Blood Flow for Strength and Hypertrophy 113
- Practical Application 113
- Final Thoughts 114

Building Bottom End Power 115
- Wide Grip Bench Presses 115
- Cambered Bar Bench Presses 117
- Dumbbell Bench Presses 119
- Bottom End Drives 120
- Final Thoughts 120

Take Home Points 121

About the Author

Josh Bryant is a speed, strength, and conditioning coach. Josh trains some of the strongest and most muscular athletes in the world in person at Metroflex Gym in Arlington, Texas, and via the Internet. Along with his receiving ISSA certifications in fitness training, nutrition, and conditioning, Josh was recently awarded the prestigious title of Master of Fitness (MFS) by the ISSA. He also has a Master's degree in Exercise Science. Josh has won many national and world titles in powerlifting and strongman and was the youngest person in powerlifting history, at 22, to bench press 600 pounds raw. Josh has squatted 909 pounds in the USPF, officially bench pressed 620 pounds raw, and officially deadlifted 800 pounds raw.

To learn more about Josh Bryant or to sign up for his free training tips newsletter, visit www.JoshStrength.com. You can also follow Josh on Twitter @JoshStrength or on Facebook/TheJoshStrengthMethod.

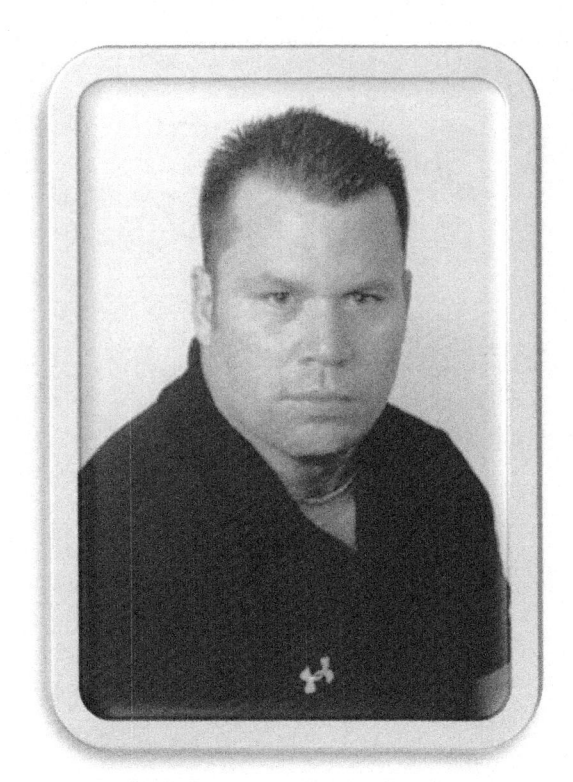

Josh Bryant - the Author

Josh is available for online training, consultations, and seminars. To learn more, visit www.JoshStrength.com.

The Bench Press

Recreational lifters and anyone sporting a semblance of a muscular physique are regularly cross-examined by friends and strangers alike on how much they can bench press.

A big bench press is your manhood in high school; it is how white collar workers assess strength, and, in some cases, it serves as an initiation tool for prison gangs. Few things are as coveted as a Herculean bench press.

Athletes and coaches place a premium on a big bench as it showcases upper body strength, tests shoulder joint integrity, and requires the fortitude to complete a grinding lift with a load capable of crushing the person beneath the bar. Powerlifters are most concerned with a bigger bench press as it drives up their three lift total.

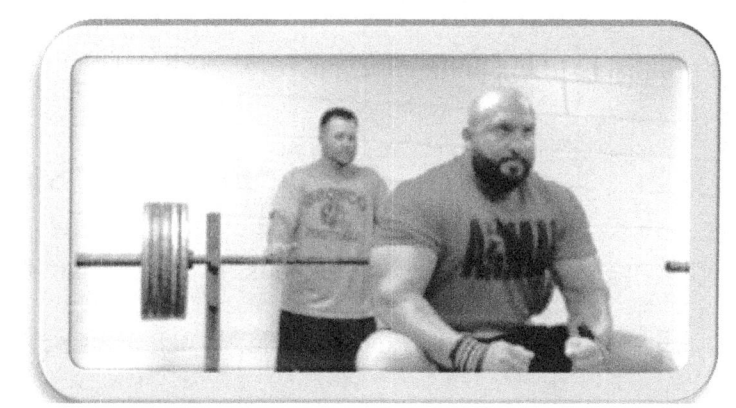

Champion Raw Powerlifter BJ Whitehead getting ready to bench press

Bodybuilders and those with physique oriented goals know that a bigger bench equates to a larger, rounder, fuller chest as well as shoulder and triceps muscles.

Even if you aren't an athlete or have any aspirations of becoming a powerlifter or bodybuilder, building a bigger bench press will arm you with bragging rights at your local gym and possibly rouse your competitive juices to step on the platform one day.

My Love Affair with the Bench Press

I have a tender spot in my heart for the bench press. I was the youngest person ever to bench press 600 pounds raw, and my methods have produced a number of lifters who have eclipsed the 600 pound mark. I will outline the methods I've created which have propelled seasoned lifters to uncharted levels of strength.

Nearly every coach with some clout can compile a who's who list of clients. Presently, I am working with a team of accomplished bench pressers, including "Big Al" Davis, Jeremy Hoornstra, Vince Dizenzo, Robert Wilkerson, and Brandon Braner. There are scores of other lifters I've worked with that have since retired, such as the legendary Ben Graves and a number of promising lifters in the pipeline.

Five "Bench Big" Strategies

Before we dive into the rest of the book, I want to share five proven strategies that have helped my clients and myself develop unrivaled bench press prowess.

1. Practice Compensatory Acceleration Training (CAT). CAT is lifting your submaximal weight with maximal force. By building explosive power in the bench press, you can blast through sticking points. Lifting the weight with the intention of being explosive will make the weight feel lighter. Need proof? Walk over to the dumbbell rack, pick up a 50-pound dumbbell quickly, and then lift it slowly. The weight will feel lighter when picked up quickly. You can't intentionally lift a maximal weight slowly.

2. Implement Dead Benches Into Your Routine. A dead bench is done in a power rack. The weight starts at chest level and is pressed up as explosively as possible. You will not be able to lift as much weight this way because of the absence of elastic-like energy stored

on the negative portion of the lift. Because of this, you will develop tremendous starting strength off the chest.

3. Do More Sets With Fewer Reps When Training For A One-Rep Max. Let's compare two prospective workouts. In Workout 1, you do 8 sets of 3 reps. Workout 2, you do 3 sets of 8 reps. In both workouts, you completed 24 repetitions; however, in Workout 1, you had 8 first reps and in Workout 2, you only had 3 first reps. Since you are training for a one-rep max, first reps are important.

4. Work Your Arms. Very few men with spaghetti arms bench press huge weights. Obviously, the triceps are crucial to lock the weight out and can be built through close-grip bench, board presses, various extensions, and a plethora of other exercises. However, the biceps help stabilize heavy weights and strong forearms help you squeeze the bar tightly. This will make the weight feel lighter in your hand. The old adage "curls are for girls" doesn't apply when it comes to moving heavy pig iron on movements such as the bench press.

5. Visualize Your Success. Your central nervous system isn't adept in differentiating between a real experience and an imagined one. Set some time aside every day to visualize yourself blasting maximal weights. Go to the gym, load your goal weight on the bar, stare at it, and envision yourself lifting it. The more vivid the experience, the more real it is. When you eventually attempt the weight, you will only be going through the motions because you have done it over and over in your head.

Be wary of when keyboard strength coaches eschew the bench press, citing it as ineffective and lacking functionality. Usually, their egos are clouding their judgment, the same egos that were

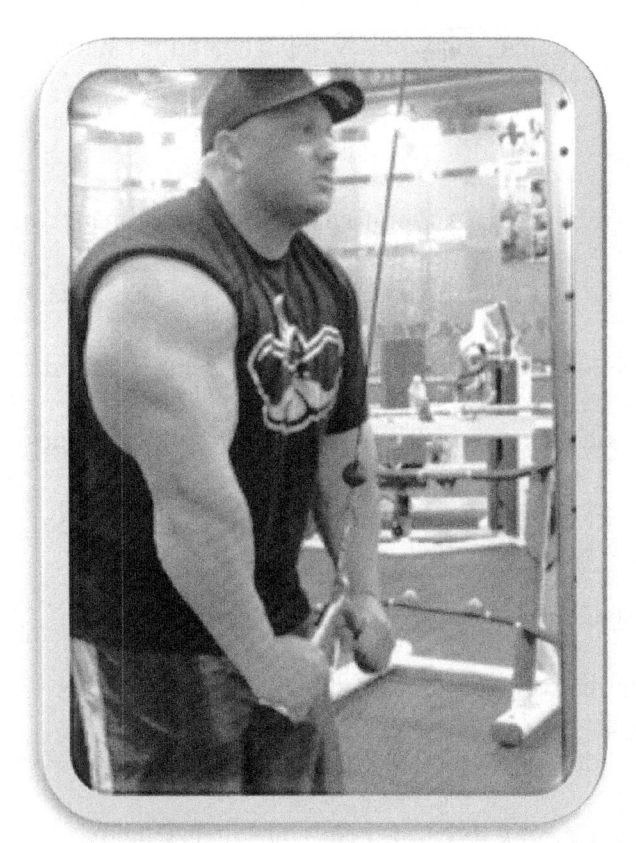

Look at the arms on Eric Spoto. Eric has bench pressed more than any human.

once humiliated when they were stapled on the bench press by a lightly loaded barbell when they began lifting. Keep in mind, those that are not good at something are generally the first to decry it.

Raw and Equipped Bench Pressing

Raw bench pressing means to limit bench press supportive equipment to a belt and wrist wraps. If you have heard about bench press world records increasing drastically since the mid-1980s, it is primarily because of the bench press shirt.

The legendary late Pat Casey first bench pressed 600 pounds in 1967. This was performed raw with Pat weighing over 300 pounds. Today, the world record raw for super heavyweights is held by Eric Spoto, with a 722-pound raw lift, set earlier this year. Only three people have ever bench pressed over 700 pounds raw, and only a select few have bench pressed over 600 pounds raw.

Progression of the Bench Press World Record

Year	Record	Gear
1898	George Hackenschmidt bench presses 361 lbs (164.09 kg).	Raw
1916	Joe Nordquest bench presses 363 lbs (165 kg).	Raw
1950s	Doug Hepburn becomes the first man to bench press 400, 450, and 500 pounds. In November 1950, he pressed 400 lbs (181.82 kg). He pressed 450 lbs (204.55 kg) in 1951, and 500 lbs (227.27 kg) in December 1953.	Raw
1959	Bruno Sammartino presses 565 lbs (256.82 kg).	Raw
1967	Pat Casey presses 615.5 lbs (279.2 kg) on March 25, 1967 and becomes the first man to bench press over 600 lbs.	Raw
1971	Jim Williams bench presses 635 lbs (288.64 kg) at the Eastern USA Open. Then, in November, he bench presses 661 lbs (300.45 kg).	Raw
1972	Jim Williams bench presses 675 lbs (306.82 kg) with only ace bandages on his elbows, wearing a t-shirt on November 9th, at the 1972 AAU World Powerlifting Championships.	Raw
1985	Ted Arcidi is the first man to bench press over 700 lbs, with a lift of 705.5 lbs (320.01 kg). This was performed in one of the first prototype supportive bench press shirts, which was 50% polyester, 50% cotton, and only one layer thick.	Shirt
1990	Ted Arcidi bench presses 718.1 lbs (325.72 kg) at the APF Bench Press Invitational on September 30 in Keene, New Hampshire.	Shirt
1993	Anthony Clark bench presses 725 lbs (329.55 kg) in May, and then in September that year, breaks his own record with a 735 lbs (334.09 kg) bench press at the USPF Northwest Open.	Shirt
1995	Jamie Harris bench presses 740 lbs (336.36 kg) at the APF State Championships.	Shirt
1998	Anthony Clark bench presses 775 lbs (351.53 kg).	Shirt
1999	Tim Isaac is the first man to bench press over 800 lbs** with a lift of 802 lbs (364.55 kg) on July 24 in Phoenix, Arizona.	Shirt
2003	Gene Rychlak is the first man to bench press 900 lbs (409.09 kg).	Shirt
2004	Gene Rychlak is the first man to bench press over 1000 lbs with a lift of 1004 lbs (456.36 kg) in November.	Shirt
2006	Scot Mendelson bench presses 1008 lbs (458.18 kg) (February 18) in a powerlifting exhibition called FIT EXPO in Pasadena, CA.	Shirt
2006	Gene Rychlak bench presses 1010 lbs (459.09 kg) (December 16).	Shirt
2007	Ryan Kennelly bench presses 1036 lbs (470.91 kg) (September 22–23).	Shirt
2007	Ryan Kennelly bench presses 1050 lbs (476.27 kg) (December 1).	Shirt
2008	Ryan Kennelly bench presses 1070 lbs (485.34 kg) (April 12).	Shirt
2008	Ryan Kennelly bench presses 1074.8 lbs (487.5 kg) (July 13).	Shirt
2008	Ryan Kennelly bench presses 1075.0 lbs (487.6 kg) (November 8).	Shirt

(http://en.wikipedia.org/wiki/Progression_of_the_bench_press_world_record)

As shirts were added to the equation and improved in supportive capabilities, records skyrocketed. The original Inzer Blast shirt, the first supportive bench press shirt on the market, added approximately 20-30 pounds to a lifter's raw bench press max. Today, there have been numerous cases of bench press shirts adding 400-500 pounds to a lifter's raw max. Physiologically, it doesn't make sense that the equipped bench press record is higher than the world record in the deadlift. In reality, the true bench press record is 300 pounds less than the world record in the deadlift. It's the equipment that's making the difference.

Progression of the Raw Bench Press World Record

Year	Record	Gear
1898	Georg Hackenschmidt bench presses 361 lbs (164.09 kg).	Raw
1916	Joe Nordquest bench presses 363 lbs (165 kg).	Raw
1950s	Doug Hepburn becomes the first man to bench press 400, 450, and 500 pounds. In November 1950 he pressed 400 lbs (181.82 kg). He pressed 450 lbs (204.55 kg) in 1951, and 500 lbs (227.27 kg) in December 1953.	Raw
1959	Bruno Sammartino bench presses 565 lbs (256.82 kg).	Raw
1967	Pat Casey bench presses 615.5 lbs (279.2 kg) on March 25, 1967 and becomes the first man to bench press over 600 lbs	Raw
1971	Jim Williams bench presses 635 lbs (288.64 kg) at the Eastern USA Open. Then, in November, he presses 661 lbs (300.45 kg).	Raw
1972	Jim Williams bench presses 675 lbs (306.82 kg) with wraps on his elbows, wearing a t-shirt on November 9th, at the 1972 AAU World Powerlifting Championships. (Not truly raw because of elbow wraps)	Raw
1996	James Henderson bench presses 705 lbs raw in a t-shirt without wrist wraps or a belt to become the first man to bench press over 700 lbs raw in May, 1996.	Raw
1997	James Henderson first bench presses 699.97 lbs, and on a later attempt the same day, 711 lbs (322.5 kg) raw without wrist wraps or a belt on July 13, 1997 at the USPF Senior Nationals in Philadelphia, Pennsylvania.	Raw
2003	Scot Mendelson bench presses 713 lbs (323.4 kg) on February 08, 2003.	Raw
2005	Scot Mendelson bench presses 715 lbs (324.3 kg) with only a belt and wrist wraps at the New England Bench Press Classic on May 22, 2005 in Worcester, Massachusetts for the highest bench press of all time without a bench press shirt.	Raw
2013	Eric Spoto bench presses 722 lbs (327.5 kg) on My 19, 2013 at an SPF Meet held at Supertraining Gym, Sacramento, CA.	Raw

(http://en.wikipedia.org/wiki/Progression_of_the_bench_press_world_record)

Progression of Records

In 1968, Bob Beamon set the world record in the long jump with a leap of 29'2.5''. To date, no one has jumped 30 feet. World records in every sport are increasing because of a larger pool of athletes, advanced training methods, and, of course, higher standards.

A 260-pound bench press increase from 1995 to 2004 is not a "natural" evolutionary sporting improvement. The raw bench press did not follow this "unnatural" improvement trend. In the late 1950s, steroids arrived on the scene. That's why the bench press jumped nearly 75 pounds at a rapid rate. Drugs have had a comparatively miniscule effect on bench press records compared to supportive shirts!

Pandora's Box Opened

By the late 1980s, elite bench pressers were rumored to be getting over 50 pounds of "help" from supportive shirts. By the 1990s, over 100 pounds of "help" was not uncommon among elite bench pressers.

During the early 2000s, bench press poundages grew at an exponential rate. Up until that point, Inzer Advanced Designs had a patent on the bench press shirt. Once other companies started producing shirts, the race was on! Within a year, it was not uncommon for lifters to routinely have lifts inflated by hundreds of pounds.

Raw Bench Pressers Physiques

While I am not advocating throwing on board shorts, getting a spray tan and entering a men's physique contest, I would be lying if I said looking good isn't important.

Look at the best raw bench pressers in the world right now: Jeremy Hoornstra and Al Davis. They look like off-season bodybuilders. Eric Spoto's physique evokes "power." By contrast, at first glance, many equipped lifters look like the only training they have been doing is at the International House of Pancakes.

Here is why bench press shirts mechanically assist lifters: elastic-like energy is stored in the supportive shirts on the eccentric/downward portion of the lift. A spring load rubber band-like effect helps catapult the weight back up to the starting position.

Supportive shirts are essentially doing the work of your muscles!

Bench press shirts are not cheating; they just don't accurately assess strength. Competing raw in an equipped contest is analogous to bringing a knife to a gun fight. Choose one or the other, and train accordingly.

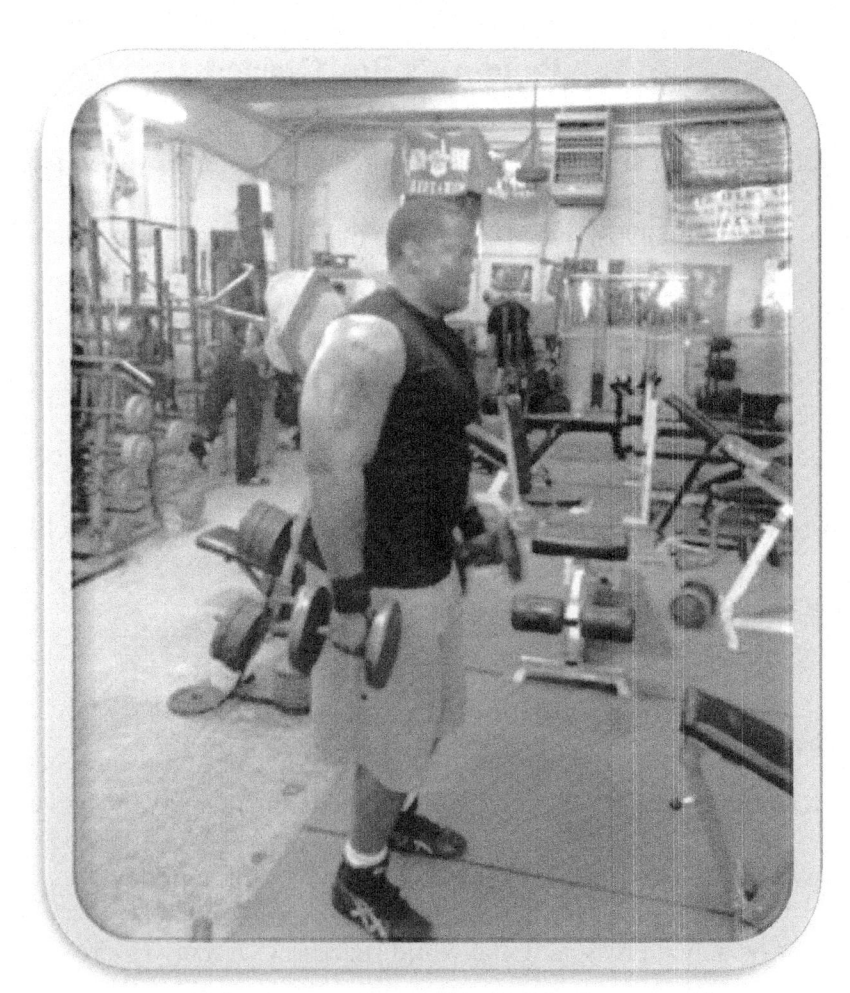

Al Davis warming up his 22.5 inch guns with light dumbbell bicep curls

If you want to learn about shirted bench pressing, there are plenty of great resources online. The intention of this book isn't to denounce shirted bench presses, but rather to looking at the science of building a huge raw bench press.

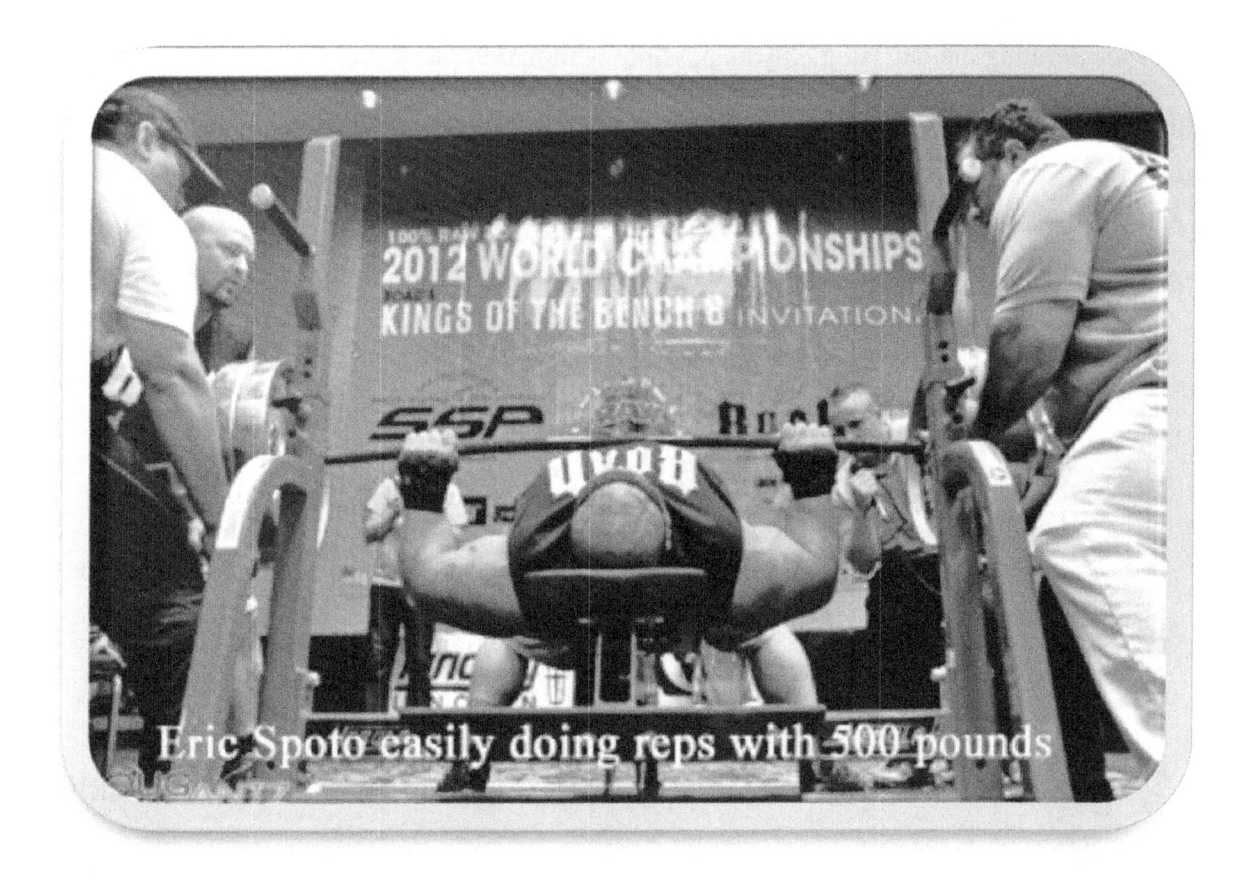

Eric Spoto easily doing reps with 500 pounds

Final Thoughts

I am going to cover methods I have used to produce multiple 600 + pound raw bench pressers and all-time world records. We are also going to take a look at the latest science on the bench press and how it is practically applicable to you and your training goals, and we will do so in layman's terms.

If you want to bench big, keep reading!

Compensatory Acceleration Training (CAT)

If lifting a barbell is a war, the central nervous system (CNS) is the general that directs that attack: accelerating the bar as quickly as possible with maximum force.

Lifting a submaximal weight with maximal force will provide many of the strength training adaptations of lifting maximal weights; on the same token, lifting a maximal weight with intent to move it as quickly as possible provides explosive strength benefits. Bottom line: your body adapts, in a large part, to your CNS's intent to move weight as rapidly as possible with maximum force.

This is Compensatory Acceleration Training, the brain child of ISSA co-founder, Dr. Fred Hatfield.

By using this technique during each rep and set, you can maximize training adaptations.

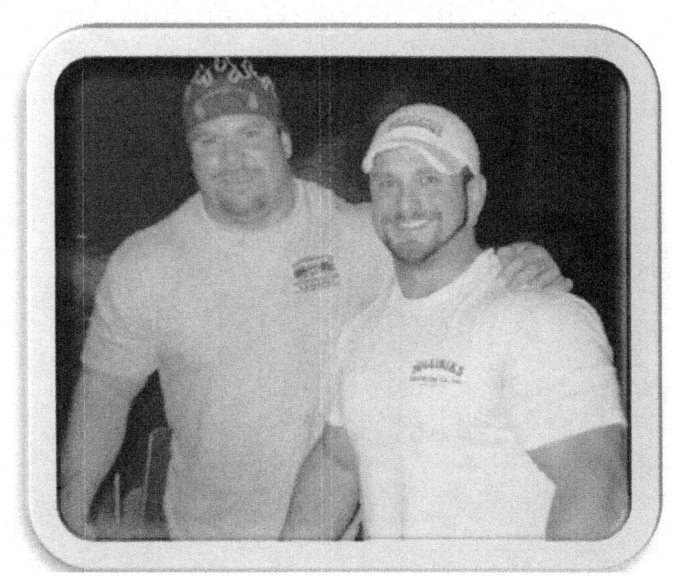

Author Josh Bryant and client Jeremy Hoornstra at 2005 Atlantis Strongest Man in America Contest

You can five board press more than you can competition bench press. During a full range of motion bench press, you have two options as leverage improves: hit the gas and accelerate the weight or put on the breaks and ride cruise control.

Compensatory Acceleration Training (CAT) means you hit the gas! In other words, you compensate for improved leverage by accelerating the weight.

From a common sense stand point, do you think you get more out a workout if you force your muscles to produce maximal force through a partial rep or the whole thing? Unless you train to get weak, small, or slow, it's the entire range of motion!

Dr. Fred Hatfield says, "Slamming a weight to the end point in the range of motion certainly would cause injury. The "learning curve" involved in slowing the movement down just before lockout is very small. Anyone can learn how to do it on the first try. It should never be a problem."

Lifting Heavy Weights Slowly?

It is impossible to lift a maximum weight with intention of moving it slowly!

Often, I am asked how to build speed in the squat, bench press, or deadlift. My response is redirecting the question back at the person on their intent when lifting the barbell. Dollars to donuts says the response will be a timid, "I just try to get the weight back up."

Hog wash!!! If you want to dominate the pig iron, you have to lose this dominated response.

Field Test

I am not expecting blind adherence to anything I am saying, I have provided a field test for you to make your decision.

Walk over to a dumbbell rack and slowly pick up a 50-pound dumbbell. Now, snatch that same dumbbell off the rack. Take note of what feels lighter?

Lifting the dumbbell fast makes it feel lighter and gives you a feeling of domination. The same holds true with a heavy barbell.

Kaz Sheds Light

In a conversation with Bill Kazmaier seven years ago about the bench press, Kaz described what he envisioned before bench pressing, "I see a big explosion going off, blowing things up. The same way I will blow the weight up. I lift it up as fast as possible." Was Kaz arguably the strongest man of all-time because he found a training program that worked for him and had great genetics? Partially, but that's only part of the scoop.

I believe what really set Kaz apart was his mindset. When Kaz bench pressed, his INTENTION was to move the weight as explosively as possible.

CAT Practically Applied

CAT is most often applied to sub maximal weights (50-80 percent of your 1RM), but the same explosive intent has to be applied to maximum weights.

Performing a max effort bench press requires maximum force production in the bottom portion of the lift, but as you lock the weight out, your ability to produce force increases. If your max is 400 pounds in the bench press, 400 pounds in your weakest range of motion will require 100 percent effort, causing adaptive overload.

However, in your strongest portion of the lift most lifters as they approach lockout, may be able to produce 600 pounds of force. As the lift becomes easier, because of increased leverage, the natural inclination is to halt maximum force production and take a free ride home. Our goal is not energy conservation! It is the training effect throughout the entire range of motion, and this can only be accomplished with Compensatory Acceleration Training.

As leverage improves, lay off cruise control and compensate by ramping up force production. This is Compensatory Acceleration Training.

By fighting your bodies' built in inhibition mechanism and maximally pushing weights as hard and fast as possible, you provide a huge overload. This is why CAT is so effective. The factors that neurologically bar you from super-human feats of strength are like bullies, continually kick and beat 'em down with CAT and they go away!

Learning to Explode

When I first started training Al Davis (670 competition raw bench press), I kept telling him to make a conscious effort to explode the weight. By the third session, he had it down. The day after Al performed CAT bench presses, Al text messaged me that his biceps were sore. This is what we are after!

C'mon, sore biceps via explosive bench pressing? Bizarre, no? The modus operandi is by locking the weight out while bench pressing, the triceps are the prime mover and the biceps are the opposing muscle acting to prevent elbow hyperextension.

The biceps serve as OSHA for explosive bench presses, regulating safety as they spare the elbow of forces associated with valgus

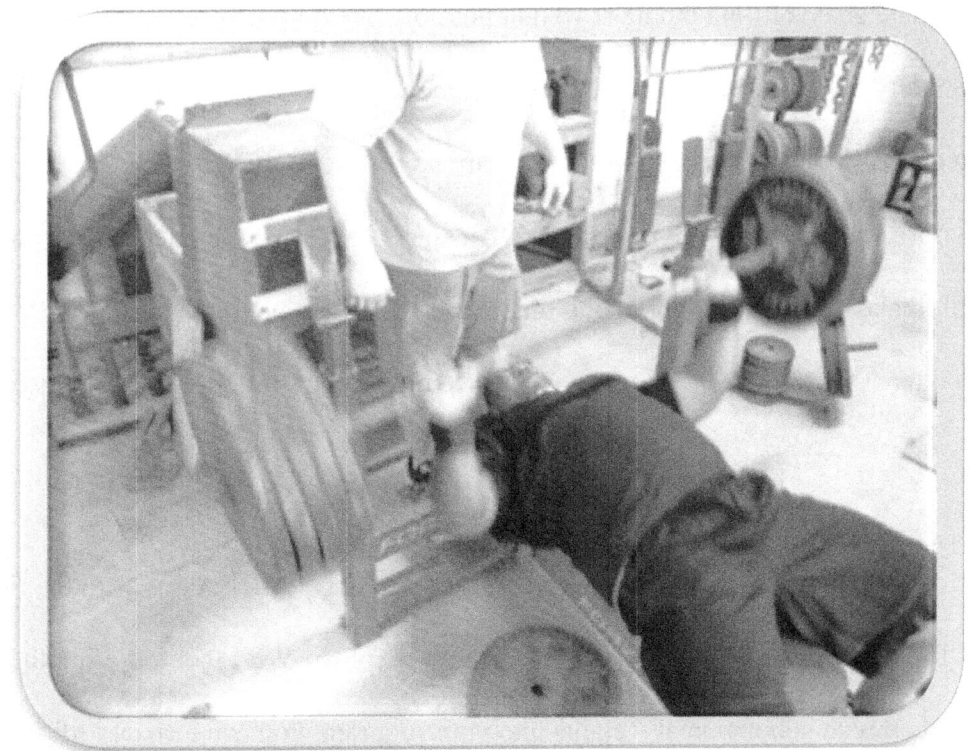

Big Al Davis CAT Bench Presses

extension overload of the elbows. The problem is, the biceps begin regulating safety way too early and limit force production capabilities. To inhibit this limiting effect, you need to train in a Compensatory Acceleration style.

Bottom line: Sore biceps following bench pressing means you reached a new realm of explosive power.

Muscle/Movement Intention Contrasted

Bodybuilders talk about muscle intention, meaning feeling the muscles working that you are targeting. For example, performing a bicep curl, you feel the biceps do the work.

I am going to introduce to you a concept I call "movement intention." This simply means when performing a core barbell movement on the concentric (positive) portion of the rep, you explode as hard as possible.

Make no attempt at selective muscle fiber recruitment; just explode as hard as possible. The ultimate goal is lifting the most weight possible; the only way to do this is simultaneously recruit as many motor units as possible by lifting the weight as explosively as possible! Ten men beat two men in tug of war, and motor units are no different.

Before you get over analytical about what special exercises you need to use to increase a certain lift, make sure you are employing this concept of movement intention. Then, and only then, will you have the knowledge to know what special exercises will be able to help you.

Any Lift Can Be Explosive

Most people don't think of bench press as an explosive lift, but it is with the right strategy.

"The truth of the matter is that any lift can be explosive! By incorporating the dynamic effort method with sub maximal weights into your program, you can turn any lift into an 'explosive' lift." Words of wisdom from top sports performance coach, Joe Defranco, who goes on to explain, "By training with weights that represent 50–60 percent of your 1RM (one rep max) in a given lift, science has proven that the weight is heavy enough to produce adequate force, yet light enough to produce adequate speed. And we should all know that speed X strength = power."

If you want to lift big weights in contests, you have to train explosively. The idea is putting maximal force in the bar each rep and each work set. In other words, do the heavy weights like they are light and the light weights like they are heavy.

To reiterate: Compensatory Acceleration Training, or CAT, is nothing more than explosive training. CAT is best done in the 55-82.5 percent range where the amount of power generated is greatest. In order to perform CAT, you must eccentrically lower the weight in a normal controlled fashion. Once you hit the bottom of the lift, very quickly change directions and explosively move the weight upward as rapidly as possible.

I remember Fred Hatfield talking about the efficiency and training effect of CAT citing squats. Even though Fred squatted 1,014 pounds, he rarely trained over 800 pounds but always applied maximum force against the bar!

CAT Efficiency

Let's say next bench press workout you will be doing five sets of four reps. If you are training like most folks, you come out of the bottom forcefully but as leverage improves, you flip on cruise control and coast to the finish.

Training in that manner severely hinders gains, look how.

> Set 1 - No bench presses were heavy enough to stimulate any sort of overload that lead to strength or power gains. Zero out of five reps provided adaptive overload, that's a zero percent efficiency rating.
>
> Set 2 - The bottom half of the last rep required enough intensity to induce some overload. Half out of five reps produced an adaptive overload, that's a 10 percent efficiency rating for true strength gains .5/5.
>
> Set 3 - The same as Set 2.
>
> Set 4 - The bottom half of the last two bench presses produced adaptive overload. Two halves equal one whole. This set has an efficiency rating of 20 percent, 1/5.
>
> Set 5 - The bottom half of all five reps produced adaptive overload. Five halves equal two and a half, still only a 50 percent efficiency rating.

Your bench press session consisted of 20 total repetitions and only nine halves produced stimulation for adaptive overload or, in other words, actually helped you get stronger. Nine halves is 4.5. 4.5 out of 20 is 22.5 percent, that's a pretty poor efficiency rating! Some gains can be made training this way but they will stagnate quicker and will never be maximized.

What if all twenty reps were bench pressed with maximal force? You'd be a heck of a lot stronger over time. You have to produce force to lift a barbell, force is mass x acceleration, and so even lifting submaximal weight quickly you can produce maximal force with less weight and less strain on your CNS.

Further CAT Benefits

At hardcore gyms, top-level pro bodybuilders routinely get out benched by guys with a lot less muscle. Sure, all else being equal, a bigger muscle will lift more. Strength is a product of the

CNS's ability to recruit and drive that muscle. This is magnified with movement intention and CAT. These higher activation limits reduce the effects of the antagonist (opposing muscles); in other words, the prime movers can do their job of lifting more weight.

Not only are you teaching your CNS to recruit more help to get the job done, but you are increasing limit strength by default via shutting down inhibitory mechanisms.

The size principle tells us muscle fibers are recruited from slow to fast. CAT can expedite the process, increasing firing frequency and fast twitch recruitment.

Furthermore, CAT increases inter and intra muscular tension, meaning muscles will more effectively work together and greater amounts of tension can be developed in individual muscles. So yes, CAT can benefit the bodybuilder.

CAT Guidelines

- Perform more sets and fewer reps-24 reps performed for eight sets of three reps is superior to three sets of eight reps for limit strength gains. Limit strength is expressed in a one rep max. More sets give more "first reps" and fewer reps allow the lifter to more easily focus on bar speed.

- Heavy weight or light weight-The intent is to move the weight as explosively as possible. The biggest fast twitch muscle fibers need to hop on board ASAP.

- Never perform CAT without warming up - Warm up sets should not be performed in a CAT style.

- Control the eccentric/explode on the concentric-This is not a super slow negative but perform the eccentric under control.

> Technique, Technique, Technique!-If technique is altered to try and move a weight faster, it won't carry over to the heavy weights. Andy Bolton, quite possibly the greatest deadlifter of all time, says, "We must stress that speed must never be at the expense of tension." In other words, stay tight and learn technique before you focus on speed.

> Perform a heavy set first-You will be more explosive because of Post-Activation Potentiation (PAP effect). Yuri Verhoshansky explains it like this, "When you perform a 3-5 RM followed by a light explosive set…to your nervous system it's like "lifting a ½ can of water when you think its full."

Let's take a look at what science has to say.

Speed - the Name of the Game

The goal in the bench press is to push the weight off your chest as quickly as possible. The sticking point results from the initial velocity of the barbell decreasing. The sticking point may be a bump in the road on the way to lockout or cause failure.

One study found that sticking points don't peak their ugly heads until 90 percent or greater of your one repetition max is eclipsed. Another study affirmed the obvious - that a sticking point is the result of not producing enough force to overcome the weight. Another study concluded sticking points are the result of a lack of transitional phases within the bench press, not because of a specific muscle group weakness.

This study consisted of subjects that had minimally one year of bench press experience. Bench presses were performed raw and compliant with strict powerlifting rules. Subjects were required to lift their max bench press and add 5.5 pounds after each successful attempt. In terms of timing, successful attempts had an average lowering phase of .97 seconds and failures were lowered faster for an average of .73 seconds.

The take home point in this study was that failure in the bench press can occur within a sticking point or even after a sticking point. Of the 11 subjects, only five failed within their sticking point, six failed subsequently.

The scientists concluded that people need to go against the traditional practice of directly addressing sticking points and focus on explosive power off the chest and carrying that speed all the way to lockout. Additionally, scientists found if you have better control on the way down, the weight is more likely to go up!

Bench Press Failure: New research indicates the sticking point is of minor concern in bench press failures. (2010). *Journal of Pure Power*, **5**

Practical Application

This confirms what I have been talking about all along. When it comes to the raw bench press, speed off the chest is the gospel. I am trying to spread that message Billy Graham style! Sticking points do not exist with enough speed off your chest. One is able to systematically bypass sticking points with enough speed. Build speed by compensatorily accelerating weights, wide grip bench presses, dead bench presses, modified cambered bar work and bench presses with bands and chains.

Sticking points can be a result of a lack of transitional phases. Think about all of the board press and partial champions out there that, when it comes to a full range of motion, can't press their way out of a paper bag. Using full range of motion, with additional bands or chains, offer the happy medium.

The Race is on with the Sticking Point

Muscle activity during the upward bench press movement was examined in this study. The researchers broke the positive into three phases:

Phase 1 - (pre-sticking point): was from the bottom of the movement until maximal barbell velocity was reached.

Phase 2 - The second period (sticking point) was from maximal barbell velocity to the barbell's lowest velocity.

Phase 3 - The period when the barbell accelerated again after the sticking point to the completion of the lift.

This study revealed that the pecs and deltoids increased activity significantly after the sticking point and when the barbell began to accelerate. The biceps decreased activity after the sticking point.

Data showed that the sticking point started .2 seconds after the initial upward movement of the barbell. Another study showed the sticking point in elite lifters was reached .35 seconds after the initial upward thrust of the barbell. All of the subjects in this study had a strength training back ground that included the bench press.

Researchers concluded that muscle activity in the prime movers decreased during the sticking point and believed this resulted from a delayed neural process. The delay may be a result of a point where the elastic-like effects of the stretch shortening cycle wear off and muscles have to fully take over. In other words, the free ride is over. If you want to keep on trucking the weight to lockout, hit the gas!

van den Tillaar, R., & Ettema, G. (2010). The "sticking period" in a maximum bench press. *Journal of Sports Sciences*, 28(5), 529-535.

Practical Application

From recreational gym rats to the cream of the crop, there is a simple take home lesson: the sticking point is reached between .2 seconds and .35 seconds after the barbell is pushed off the chest. Power out of the gate is gospel! You cannot lift a heavy weight slow. Explosive bench pressing power is built through strategies outlined throughout the book with Compensatory Acceleration Training (CAT) being the bread and butter.

Light has also been shed on the importance of bench press specific plyometrics. Plyometrics enhance the stretch shortening cycle; in other words, you get better at storing elastic-like energy to spring the bar off your chest. If the sticking point results from this spring-like effect being dissipated, we have to maximize this spring-like effect!

The spring-like effect can be maximized with CAT bench presses, plyometrics and bottom end drives. The advanced lifter wanting to amplify this effect can add bands.

Because the sticking point hits within a third of a second or less, starting strength must be trained hard if you want to bench press big raw. This is done with dead benches, deep dumbbell pause benches, cambered bar bench presses, wide grips and other strategies discussed throughout the book.

Because deltoid and chest activity are increased as you push through the sticking point, it is important to train these muscles; it will require more than just bench pressing. Since the 1990s, shirted "guru's" have expressed a condescending tone toward chest and deltoid isolation exercises like flys and front raises, totally dismissing the fact that pretty much every great raw bench presser has included these in their regimen. Only recently have some of these folks started to warm up toward overhead press.

Man cannot live off the bench press alone! You have to work some "bodybuilding" movements to directly hit the muscles involved. Remember, a chain is as strong as its weakest link. Bench press will always be the core of your bench press program. If your chest is the weak link, it will not get sufficient stimulation from bench press alone because of synergistic dominance or assisting muscles doing the job of the pecs. Furthermore, bench pressing requires a focus on performing the movement as explosively as possible, not on contracting individual muscles, so some isolation work is needed.

In summary, as lifters move past the sticking point, bicep activity significantly decreases. This is because as a lifter locks the weight out the biceps are the opposing muscle to the prime mover, the triceps. Because of reciprocal inhibition, or a relaxation of the biceps, the triceps can do their job and bicep activity decreases. The faster the biceps relax, the faster we can lock the weight out. We can train the inhibitory effect of the biceps and the golgi tendon organ (GTO) by training explosively in a CAT style, using bands and chains and, of course, the implementation of bench press specific plyometrics.

Compensatory Acceleration Training (CAT) Reigns Supreme

Okay, so this "CAT" idea sounds great, but what does science say? Glad you asked. This study examined the effects on strength after training for three weeks of the bench press with maximal speed (CAT) and a self-selected slower pushing speed. There were 20 total subjects, 10 trained in a CAT style on the bench press, the other half with a self-selected speed. Both groups trained with 85 percent of their one repetition max twice a week.

Prior to the commencement of training and after cessation of the three weeks of training, pushing speed and one repetition max were measured. The group that trained in a CAT style increased their bench press speed by 2.2 percent and strength by 10.2 percent, the self-selected group showed no improvements in either category.

Padulo, J. J., Mignogna, P. P., Mignardi, S. S., Tonni, F. F., & D'Ottavio, S. S. (2012). Effect of different pushing speeds on bench press. *International Journal of Sports Medicine*, 33(5), 376-380.

Practical Application

This again is one more study confirming the importance of explosive power in the raw bench press. CAT style is required to continually ellicit gains in the bench press in trained subjects. I have seen this happen many times. Once an athlete, regardless of experience, learns to truly bench press with max force, strength goes through the roof. To reach your maximum strength levels in the bench press, you have to train in a compensatory acceleration style.

Lifting Maximal Weight Increase Force Production in Subsequent Sets

Post Activation Potentiation (PAP) is a strategy used to improve performance in power activities and refers to the enhancement of muscle function following a high force activity. Legendary Russian Sports Scientist Yuri Verhoshansky explained PAP in layman's terms as follows, "When you perform a 3-5 Rep Max followed by a light explosive set…to your nervous system it's like lifting a ½ can of water when you think it's full." The weight feels lighter and moves faster.

This study set out to determine if power during bench press exercise was increased when preceded by one repetition maximum (1RM) in the bench press prior to lifting submaximal weights with maximal force, and it also aimed to determine the optimal rest interval to optimize PAP response.

The four experimental sessions were composed of a one repetition max followed by Compensatory Acceleration Training (CAT) sets with rest intervals consisting of 1, 3, 5, and 7 minutes, performed on different days, and determined randomly. Power was measured via peak power equipment (Cefise, Nova Odessa, São Paulo, Brazil).

The study determined there was a significant increase in PAP in concentric muscle contractions after seven minutes of recovery after a max weight was used. The results suggest that seven minutes of recovery has generated an increase in PAP in bench.

Ferreira, S., Panissa, V., Miarka, B., & Franchini, E. (2012). Postactivation Potentiation: Effect of Various Recovery Intervals on Bench Press Power Performance. *Journal of Strength & Conditioning Research* **(Lippincott Williams & Wilkins), 26(3), 739-744.**

Practical Application

I wrote about reverse pyramiding in Muscle Mag International a couple years ago. The idea is to start off with your heaviest sets, and then perform submaximal sets. This takes advantage of the PAP effect. If a football player is getting ready for a combine with a 225-pound rep bench press rep max, I will have him bench press 275-315 pounds first, the end result is he always performs more reps. "You feel like you are lifting half of a can like it's full," in Dr. Verhoshansky words. This allows you to build strength very effectively because the most important strength building set is the first set in this rep scheme. You are 100 percent fresh! What most people don't look at is the fact that you will produce greater forces on your CAT sets following your heavy sets. Many studies on PAP are generally done on things like heavy squats followed by an explosive activity like a vertical jump. Countless studies show the effectiveness of PAP, but it's cool to see what I've known and advocated for years to be validated by science. We have learned the same effect holds true when moving from a maximal weight to a sub maximal weight. In layman's terms, bench 500 first then 400 feels lighter and it will move more explosively.

CAT Training Continually Reigns Supreme

Division 1 football players training in a compensatory acceleration style (CAT) upper body strength regimen were compared to a traditional regimen in their off-season. The CAT group was instructed to perform the positive rep as explosively as possible. The traditional group performed repetitions at a traditional tempo.

At the end of both off-season training programs, both power and strength were assessed. Power was tested with a seated medicine ball throw and a force platform plyometric push-up test. Strength was assessed by a one rep max in the bench press.

Both groups increased strength and power. The group that trained in a Compensatory Acceleration Training (CAT) style improved their bench press by nearly double the amount of the traditional group. Average power, as expected, increased significantly more in the group that trained explosively.

Jones, K. K., Hunter, G. G., Fleisig, G. G., Escamilla, R. R., & Lemak, L. L. (1999). The effects of compensatory acceleration on upper-body strength and power in collegiate football players. *Journal of Strength & Conditioning Research* **(Allen Press Publishing Services Inc.), 13(2), 99-105.**

Practical Application

Fred Hatfield was ahead of his time advocating Compensatory Acceleration Training. It is simply superior! Training adaptations are not just a result of weight on the bar. Adaptations from training are a byproduct of tension and duration. You respond to how much force produced, how fast the force was produced, how long you produced it, and how many times you produced it. Force=mass x acceleration. More tension is result of greater bar speed. Maximal strength training and power adaptations can result from lifting weights with maximal force; one more reason to compensatorily accelerate weights.

Tempo and Power Output

Let's take a look at tempo for maximum strength and power acquisition. Fast negatives (one second) with no pause in the bottom position resulted in the greatest power output gains, i.e. the most explosive bench presses. When the negative was slowed down and pauses were added to the bottom position, peak power declined. Negatives of one to four seconds were contrasted. As the time of the lowering phase increased, power decreased. Lifters were additionally able to complete more repetitions with 80 percent of their one repetition maxes with a faster eccentric.

Pryor, R. R., Sforzo, G. A., & King, D. L. (2011). Optimizing Power Output By Varying Repetition Tempo. *Journal of Strength & Conditioning Research* **(Lippincott Williams & Wilkins), 25(11), 3029-3034**

Practical Application

In a powerlifting meet, you have to pause. You need to practice how you play. That's why it's important to include pause bench presses and some supplementary movements emphasizing pauses. Do not pause CAT bench presses. Pauses negate some of the benefits of the stretch shortening cycle. We need great starting strength from a dead stop. At the same time, we need to perform like spring-loaded cannons, enhancing our elastic properties derived from the SSC. Bottom line is: train both ways!!

Final Thoughts

To maximize strength gains you have to train in a CAT style. Repetition is the mother of skill. By performing rep after rep and set after set in this style, your CNS will be primed for maximal strength, rate of force development will be enhanced, neurological inhibitions will be reduced, and you will experience the greatest muscular overload.

Elimination of Sticking Points: A Scientific Approach

"I don't want to get any messages saying, 'I am holding my position.' We are not holding a damned thing. Let the Germans do that. We are advancing constantly, and we are not interested in holding onto anything, except the enemy's balls. We are going to twist his balls and kick the living shit out of him all of the time. Our basic plan of operation is to advance and to keep on advancing regardless of whether we have to go over, under, or through the enemy. We are going to go through him like crap through a goose; like shit through a tin horn!"

-General Patton

This quote from Patton's iconic speech to the Third Army is the attitude we need to have toward sticking points!

In the war on sticking points, the weapon of choice is increased bar acceleration. Push a bar fast enough, all sticking points are eliminated. Bar speed is like a nuclear bomb; it destroys sticking points in an instant.

But if you are already training in a Compensatory Acceleration Style and have mastered movement intention, you don't have a nuclear bomb to wipe out the sticking point opposition. Have no fear, as many wars have been won with superior ground troops! In the sticking point war, isometrics are superior ground troops.

The establishment preaches that isometrics have no training value, having been abandoned by knuckle draggers generations ago because of their localized strengthening effect.

The powers that be are correct on their localized strengthening assertion. But hogwash on elimination! The reasoning for this antiquated avoidance of isometrics is why we embrace them.

Think about it: As you push the weight up in the bench press, your ability to produce force will change, even decreasing in some regions. The objective is to accelerate the bar up as fast as possible. A sticking point occurs where the ability to produce force is decreased.

The localized strength gaining effects of isometrics, what the establishment calls "destructive training," is how we destroy sticking points.

Let's take a look at the lost art of isometrics, which have helped build some of the strongest men of all time!

What is an Isometric Contraction?

An isometric contraction is defined as a muscular contraction not accompanied by movement of the joint. Resistance applied to the contraction increases muscular tension without producing movement of the joint.

Isometrics could mean holding a weight in place, like a crucifix hold in a strongman contest. The goal is to not "yield" to the weight and begin an eccentric/negative contraction. In Russian literature this is referred to as a yielding contraction.

The other type of isometric contraction is lifting against an immovable object. This is what prompts the biggest strength gains and what we will focus on. When pushing against an immovable object you are able to produce 15% more force than you could dynamically in the same spot. Consequently, you are teaching your Central Nervous System to produce more force in your weakest spots. This will produce a localized strengthening effect specific to the sticky region you are targeting.

Your CNS: The Predator, Not the Prey

Holding a weight in place does not have the same effect as pushing against an immovable object. Strength is primarily a function of the central nervous system. Do you want to program your central nervous system to: A) Passively not yield to a weight or B) Prison rape your sticking points, pushing the bar into oblivion with maximal force?

I like Option B any day of the week and twice on Sunday. Don't only look at the effects on your musculature; look at the intent of your CNS. Your CNS needs to be programmed to aggressively push through sticking points. Program the CNS and the barbell and muscles follow. The CNS is the general in the strength army, your muscles are troops.

Remember when you are holding a weight in place, you are not producing maximal force!

Determining Sticking Points

In 1981, Don Pfeiffer wrote, "The proper way to determine where the sticking point occurs is to observe successful bench presses. The best method is to perform several sets of bench presses with weight that will allow 3-6 reps. Your only concern should be the successful completion of the lift, while someone watches you perform the lift to determine the sticking point. The area where the bar's ascent slows down or momentarily comes to a halt is where the sticking point occurs."

After the sticking point is determined, we can try to identify the weak link muscle. This is nearly impossible with 100 percent accuracy. The other option is to build specific strength in that area where the sticking point occurs. This is where isometrics come in.

Isometrics for the Bench Press

Isometrics are much more common on the squat and deadlift, but should be part of the bench press's sticking point elimination arsenal. Isometrics will increase your bench press when properly applied.

Potential Causes of Sticking Points

Sticking points can result from a halt of the benefits of the elastic-like energy derived from the stretch shortening cycle that helps you press the weight back up after lowering it.

If this seems complicated, try this: jump up as high as possible. Do one jump by dipping your butt down and jumping up in the air. Do the second jump without dipping your butt down, in a bottom up, squat jump fashion. You jump a lot higher dipping first. This is because of the elastic-like energy stored as you dip down. The same concept applies to the bench press. As the elastic-like energy wears off when you push the bar up, the bar will slow down.

Speed and Sticking Points

Speed is the name of the game. If you do not accelerate fast enough off your chest with the barbell, it will eventually stop and go back down. With this in mind, a recent study measured isometric force production of 12 different regions of the bench press. Force production varied at the different regions. This showed there were mechanically weak areas.

This brings us to the chief complaint against isometrics: they only develop strength in specific regions of movement. This region ranges 15 degrees from where the isometric contraction is being performed. So if the isometric contraction is being performed with your elbow bent at 90 degrees, strength adaptations will take place at 75-105 degrees of elbow flexion.

Because isometrics only provide strength gains in a limited range of motion, this is the perfect sticking point remedy. A sticking point is a weakness in a limited range of motion. To reiterate: what the naysayers forgot to tell you, is that you are capable of producing around 15 percent more force in an isometric contraction than you can in a concentric/positive contraction. You can work a specific range of motion and do it with more force.

If a sticking point is a disease, the isometric is the vaccination!

Isometrics and the PAP Effect

Maximal isometric contractions are beyond a maximal weight. It is a supramaximal weight because you can produce 15 percent more force than you could when pushing the weight up. This magnifies the PAP effect!!

After performing a maximal isometric contraction, wait 1-7 minutes and perform a submaximal set in a CAT style. The bar will literally feel like it is going to fly out of your hands! Not only will this lead to a higher force production, but it will help inhibit your body's built in safety mechanisms like the Golgi Tendon Organ (GTO.) This type of neural inhibition is the gateway to world class strength, much more important than a "pump."

Understanding Isometrics

As the old proverb goes, "Give a man a fish, feed him for a day. Teach a man to fish, feed him for life!"

Now you are starting to understand how and why isometrics work. Knowing the why will help you understand how to program these movements and how to invent your own variations.

Isometrics, World Records and Pink Pills

Isometrics were popularized by Dr. John Ziegler, the team physician for the York Barbell Club in the 1950s and 1960s. Bob Hoffman, the owner of York Barbell Club, made millions of dollars because of their training system using Isotonic-Isometrics.

Hoffman said functional isometrics will "bring superior results faster, with far less effort, in a great deal less time. It will be a body saver because its scientific method builds the maximum of strength and development, with a minimum strain upon muscles, tendons and ligaments."

The isometrics Hoffman advocated is pushing against an immovable object. For instance, the standing overhead press was a contested lift in Olympic lifting in those days. If a lifter wanted to work at the point where the bar is near his eyes, he would push with maximum force against the pins on a power rack at eye level, generally holding the contraction for six to ten seconds.

The isotonic-isometrics that Ziegler developed were different than traditional isometrics because isotonic means there is a change in muscle length. The lifter would move the bar to a specific place before pushing against the immovable object, as opposed to starting and stopping the push at the same point. Today, many refer to this as functional isometrics.

Not only were world records set by Olympic lifters, athletes using Ziegler's isometric system showed impressive results. Legendary track and field athlete Jay Sylvester repeatedly broke the world record in the discus! Jay publicly acknowledged that a large part of his success resulted from strength gains attained through isometric training.

Jim Beatty, arguably the greatest one miler ever, partially credited the world record he set in the mile to isometric training. At a time when it was considered taboo for athletes outside of competitive weightlifting to lift weights, athletes from a plethora of sports were breaking records left and right, partially crediting their success to isometric training.

Bill March, the poster boy for the isometric training system and the York Barbell Club, began breaking records in weightlifting every time he competed. March stated publicly over and over that his new found record setting strength was because of the isometric strength training system Ziegler had developed. Other lifters with record setting performances from York Barbell Club echoed March's sentiment.

This metamorphosis of isometric strength training sounds like it single handedly changed strength records, track records, and revolutionized the performance of other sports. There is more to the story, folks! Dr. Ziegler left out one detail to why his athletes were so successful! In 1954, Dr. Ziegler accompanied the York Barbell Team to the World Weightlifting Championships held in Vienna, Austria. While there, Ziegler saw the Russians dominate the event and set many records. In addition, the extremely muscular and hairy physiques of the Russians made the American weightlifters appear like boys.

This piqued Dr. Ziegler's curiosity, so he invited the Russian team physician out for a night on the town.

The story has it that as the vodka was flowing, the Russian physician became inebriated. Dr. Ziegler saw an opportunity to ask the Russian about their secret. The Russian doctor revealed that the Russians had been building strength and muscle with testosterone.

After that night, Dr. Ziegler felt that to put the Americans on an even playing field, they would have to use testosterone in their training regiments.

Bob Hoffman, coach and owner of York Barbell Club, joyfully granted Dr. Ziegler access to his team. Ziegler began to experiment straight testosterone shots to weightlifters and bodybuilders at Hoffman's club. Yet, this proved to be unsuccessful. Nonetheless, this did not discourage Ziegler in his pursuit of developing a "wonder" drug. In 1958, he partnered with Ciba

Pharmaceuticals and created Methandrostenolone, which was called Dianabol, and is referred to by some as "D-bol".

Dianabol proved to work quite well, and American weightlifters were once again competitive on the international scene. As you know, Ziegler claimed this was because of the isometric training system he had developed. However, many who used his system without Dianabol were disappointed in the results.

Once the cat was let out of the bag, folks dismissed isometrics as a useless marketing ploy by York Barbell Club to line Hoffman's pockets. While Hoffman clearly wanted to make money, it is unfair to dismiss isometric training as a useless brouhaha.

Think about how many times you have found out someone is taking steroids, yet your little brother can destroy them in the gym, on the field, or in a street fight. I can think of countless examples of people that prove the point that steroids don't make everyone a champion!

I'm not a betting man, but I'd wager that the top drug-free powerlifters will out lift 99 percent of their juiced-up counterparts. Why am I saying this? The importance of an effective training program will trump an elaborate steroid cycle almost always. If you are on the juice but train without intelligence, intensity, and guts, you will not set world records in a drug-free powerlifting meet.

The same holds true in Olympic lifting. Strength is a product of neural factors (how efficiently your CNS recruits the proper motor units) and how much muscle mass you have. Steroids enhance muscle mass but have not been conclusively shown to enhance neural factors to the same degree. Do steroids work? Absolutely! Was that the main reason Bill March, the first American to use Dianabol, made a majority of his gains? Probably! However, March would not have set world records had he trained like a moron. Isometrics clearly played an important role!

Isometric Drawbacks

Unfortunately, isometrics have fallen out of favor in strength training programs in the last half century. Isometrics should not be the core of any strength training program, unless of course, the goal of that program is to maximize isometric strength. Here are some of the potential drawbacks of isometric training.

- Isometrics are very demanding on the Central Nervous System (CNS). You are producing much larger force in isometric movements than in their dynamic counterparts and are literally exerting maximum balls out effort and force into the bar. This can/will place a tremendous strain on your CNS. Take home point: one glass of red wine a day can benefit your health; five bottles a day can destroy your health. Think of isometrics like red wine.

- The Valsalva Maneuver is when a person tries to exhale forcibly with a closed glottis (the windpipe) so that no air exits through the mouth or nose. The Valsalva maneuver impedes the return of venous blood to the heart. This causes a huge spike in blood pressure and greatly increases heart rate. A healthy person should return to resting levels quickly. If you have any type of cardiovascular issues, you are playing Russian roulette by using this technique. Even if you are healthy, you are taking a minor risk, although the risk of driving to the gym is greater. I assume by reading this book, you are after performance. Everything has a risk to benefit ratio, so be informed! Bench press specific isometrics are most effective when you use the Valsalva Maneuver. Numerous studies have shown this technique allows athletes to produce greater forces, and this technique keeps the athlete tight and produces a more rigid torso. Between sets of isometric exercises, it is recommended for the athlete to perform breathing and relaxation exercises.

- ➢ Isometrics do not allow a true quantitative measure of strength without some sort of a dynamometer. Isometrics require a true, honest, maximal effort and are not a good choice for those that lack mental toughness.

- ➢ Isometrics performed too frequently, too long, and not properly integrated with dynamic strength training exercises can decrease the rate of force development. The abuse of isometrics can inhibit the stretch-shortening cycle (ssc) by destroying the elastic properties of muscles that enhance quick, powerful, movements. This is crucial to explosive, athletic movements in sports. Remember the bench press is a reversible muscle action.

Training Benefits & Guidelines

Quoting EliteFTS.com founder and CEO, Dave Tate, "Isometrics have limited value, but limited value is some value." The better your bench press becomes, the more benefit limited value will have!

If your goal is to go from 150 pounds to 200 pounds in the bench press, nearly any sensible program will work. If you plan to increase your bench press from 500 pounds to 600 pounds, it gets complex, unless you are some sort of genetic mutant. You will need to be more and more selective in the methods of strength training you include in your regimen.

Isometrics in your routine offer some of the following benefits:

- ➢ Isometrics allow athletes to maximize their strength to bodyweight ratio. This ratio is an athlete's relative strength or limit strength (how much force an athlete can exert in one all-out effort regardless of time) divided by his bodyweight. Isometrics are one of the most effective methods to increase limit strength. Limit strength is increased primarily by two different mechanisms:

1. An increase in the area of cross-sectional muscle fiber, in other words: muscle size.
2. Secondly, by neural factors: how efficiently your nervous system can recruit the necessary motor units to produce maximal force.

➢ Isometrics enhance the second mechanism. If your goal is primarily to add size, isometrics are not the plan of action. However, isometrics reign supreme for increasing neural recruitment patterns to produce maximal force, but are inferior for muscle gains! One 2001 study showed that you are able to recruit 5 percent more motor units/muscle fibers with a maximal isometric contraction compared to an eccentric or concentric contraction. When it comes to motor unit recruitment, more is better.

➢ If you have a very limited time to train your bench press, isometric bench press training maximizes strength gains and minimizes training time. If you lift a maximal effort bench press, you will only be executing maximum force for a fraction of a second. Compare that to a five second isometric contraction against the pins. It would take exponentially more traditional bench press (dynamic movement) to equate to an equal amount of time producing maximal force when holding an isometric contraction for five seconds. Love 'em or hate 'em, but isometrics are a model of efficiency for developing a huge bench press.

- One common, simplistic complaint against using isometrics in strength training programs is they produce large strength increases, but they are increased at the joint angle they are performed, plus or minus 15 degrees. For instance, an isometric barbell curl where the elbow is 90 degrees into flexion will increase strength at a joint angle of 75 to 105 degrees but have virtually no effect at 60 degrees. The increases in strength are very, very localized! Many see this as a disadvantage and many times, it is. For instance, when a strength coach is putting a large group of athletes through a basic strength training program. For someone looking to increase their bench press at a specific sticking point, there is no better way to do it than isometrics! One man's terrorist is another man's freedom fighter. If you want the freedom to set PRs and want to terrorize and eliminate sticking points that have been holding you back, isometrics have a great value. Isometrics can be worked up to 5 points per work out. Generally, 1-3 is sufficient. Minimally, use a 10 to 1 rest to work ratio, so if you hold the contraction for 5 seconds, rest at least 50 seconds.

- Many popular training techniques nowadays require fancy equipment; if you have a power rack, a barbell and some weights, you can perform isometrics that will benefit your bench press.

- Maximum intramuscular tension is just a brief part of the M.O. for a maximum concentric. Think leverage changes, bar speed, etc. Maximal tension would be tough to maintain for even 1/3 of a second dynamically, but you can do it for 5 seconds isometrically. Think about the training economy. The maximal tension in 15 dynamic contractions can essentially be replicated in one isometric contraction. This is a very economical method.

- Improvement in starting strength and the ability to reach maximum force production rapidly.
- Isometrics must be trained with dynamic movements; isometrics supplement dynamic force production, and isometrics are a means to an end.
- Isometric gains cease after 6-8 weeks. Do not use year round.
- To maximize benefits, contract as hard as possible. If maximum intramuscular coordination is not reached, you are wasting your time.
- Isometric bench presses can help identify weaknesses. The reason is simple. It is much harder to see and identify poor lifting technique/inefficient movement patterns during a dynamic movement than during a static hold that produces maximum force.
- Isometrics have a PAP effect and can help neutrally inhibit factors that limit force production.

Quasi Isometrics

Mel Siff in his book Super Training coins the term "Quasi-Isometric Action." A quasi isometric muscle action is a dynamic maximal effort lift by an athlete. Because of the excessively heavy load, the athlete moves the load very slowly. During a true isometric, the load does not move. A very heavy, slow dynamic contraction is close to an isometric contraction, and this is why I believe Siff coined the term.

Quasi Isometric muscle actions are heavy and slow. Bench press specific isometrics will offer greater transference; the heavier the load, the more the maximal effort lift resembles a quasi isometric, and the better the transfer of training. If your goal is to increase your max bench press and overall limit strength, bench press specific isometrics certainly have a place in your bag of tricks!

The Risk to Benefit Ratio of Bench Press Specific Isometrics

Whether you are trying to meet ladies on match.com or increase your bench press, the decisions you make should be to maximize the benefit and minimize the risk. There are drawbacks to overusing isometrics. Here are some effective ways I have found to help maximize the benefits of isometrics and circumvent possible negative effects.

- Isometrics should be performed against an immovable, strong, solid structure. Don't start the isometric contraction at the point the isometric contraction will take place. Some dynamic movement is recommended pre and post contraction, the same way Bob Hoffman advocated fifty years ago. It worked then, and it works now.

- Do not exceed six seconds for isometric contractions. I recommend five seconds. It is not uncommon to hear of lifters doing these for 15 seconds. This can cause all sorts of negative effects and is unsafe. "Train for pain" is a senseless adage someone scribbled on the wall at Metroflex Gym, and this is the mentality of isometrics held too long. Remember, train for maximum results. PRs, records, titles, and results are our objectives, not silly, self-inflicted pain. Limit the total isometric portion of your training session to less than 10 percent. A good rule of thumb: If you're spending more than ten minutes of your workouts engaging in isometric training, you are abusing it.

- Perform some sort explosive dynamic work after isometric contractions for the benefit of your central nervous system and positive neural adaptations. When contrasting with a dynamic movement, the 10 minute rule no longer applies.

- Isometrics can be utilized pre competition to eliminate stubborn sticking points or off-season to target specific weaknesses.

➤ After a workout that contains isometrics, I recommend some breathing exercises, static stretching and/or PNF stretching, and some foam rolling.

Functional Isometrics

A couple years ago, legendary strength coach Charles Poliquin did a piece on isometric training. Poliquin calls his method functional isometrics. For the bench press, this method would be done inside a power rack; the lifter would put a bench in the power rack and set the pins in the power

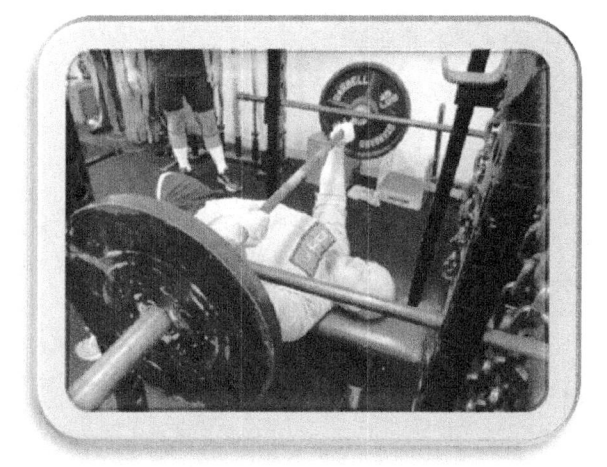

Ross Shreves at the top and bottom of a functional isometric exercise

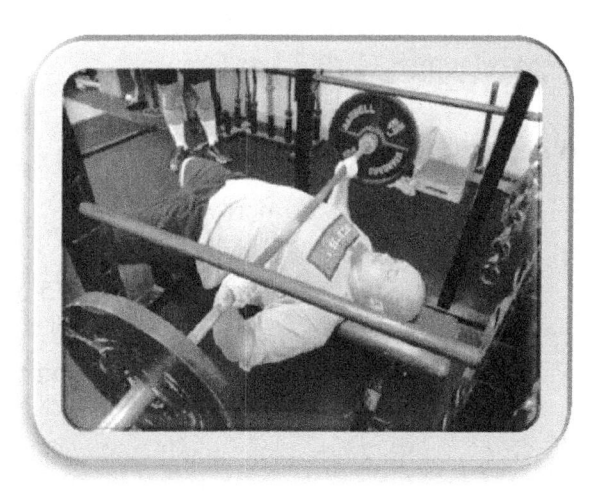

rack at the height of his sticking point. The set would start by the lifter bench pressing the barbell to the pins, just briefly touching them and returning to the starting position. This would be done for 6-8 total repetitions. On the final repetition, the lifter would push with maximal force against the pins for 6-8 seconds isometrically.

Poliquin says if you can do another rep after pushing against the pins, the weight you are using is too light. Lifters have had success with this method.

Functional Isometric Routine

Here is a practical application of this method in a four week block:

Week 1

1) Bench Press 90 percent x 2 reps

2) CAT Bench Press rest 90 seconds 75 percent x 3 reps x 4 sets

3) Functional Isometrics at sticking point x 6 reps x 3 sets

4) Chest Supported Dumbbell Rows/Chain Fly Superset 12 reps each x 3 supers

5) Band Resisted Triceps Extension 5 sets 12 reps

6) Hammer Curls 3 sets 6 reps

Week 2

1) Bench Press 92.5 percent x 2 reps

2) CAT Bench Press rest 90 seconds 75 percent x 3 reps x 5 sets

3) Functional Isometrics at sticking point x 7 reps x 3 sets

4) Chest Supported Dumbbell Rows/Chain Fly Superset 15 reps each x 3 supersets

5) Band Resisted Triceps Extensions 5 sets 10 reps

6) Hammer Curls 3 sets 8 reps

Week 3

1) Rest Paused Bench Press 95 percent (do a single rest 30 seconds, repeat, do as many singles as possible without failing)

2) CAT Bench Press rest 90 seconds 75 percent x 3 reps x 6 sets

3) Functional Isometrics at sticking point x 8 reps x 3 sets

4) Chest Supported Dumbbell Rows/Chain Fly Superset 10 reps each x 3 supersets

5) Band Resisted Triceps Extensions 5 sets 8 reps

6) Hammer Curls 3 sets 10 reps

Week 4
> Deload

Isodynamics

The scariest part of adding bench press isometrics to a traditional athlete's training regimen, particularly for a bench presser who is reliant on speed, is isometrics performed too frequently, too long and not properly integrated with dynamic strength training exercises can adversely affect the ability to rapidly develop force and retard the stretch-shortening cycle (SSC).

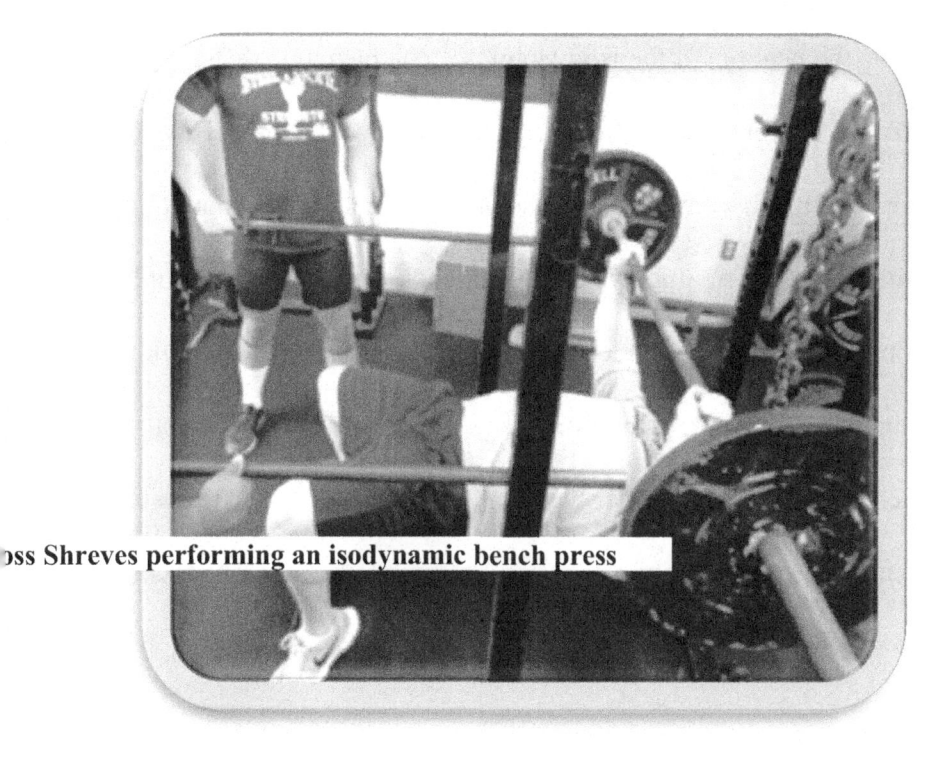

Ross Shreves performing an isodynamic bench press

Luckily, we can circumvent these adverse consequences with what I call Isodynamics. Isodynamics require two COMPETENT lifting partners. They are performed like traditional bench press isometrics (5 second hold). However, after the lifter has pushed against the immovable pins, he is not finished. Two partners, one on each side of the power rack, will very quickly pull both pins out of the rack. The lifter will then lower the weight to his chest and explosively press the weight to lockout. Because of the PAP effect from the maximal isometric contraction, along with lowering the bar back to the chest (stretch reflex), the lifter should be able to push the bar back to lockout with supramaximal force.

Mass x Acceleration =Force. Remember, we produce maximal force with approximately 60 percent of our one repetition max. For isodynamics, use 60 percent of your 1 repetition bench max. This is not important for the isometric portion of the lift, but is extremely important for the dynamic contraction because the goal is maximum force and velocity.

What if I have no competent helpers to perform Isodynamics?

Luckily for you, you can still receive the benefits of the isodynamics. You have two different options. The first one is to perform the maximal isometric contraction for five seconds. Have a loaded bar with 50 percent of your 1 rep max (we will use less so you still feel explosive, but you will not get the added benefit of the stretch shortening cycle) right outside the rack. Immediately following the isometric contraction, bench press the loaded bar with maximal force. Again, this teaches your central nervous system to explode after a maximal isometric contraction. The other option is to immediately do a bench press plyometric after the isometric bench press. The best option, besides isodynamics, is bench pressing 50 percent of your 1 rep max after the five second isometric contraction. It is more sport specific.

Isodynamic Routine

Here is a practical example of a four week block including isodynamics.

Week 1

1) Bench Press 75 percent x 1 x 15 sets (rest 30 seconds between sets, last set as many reps as possible)

2) Isodynamic (at sticking point) x 3 sets

3) Two Board Cambered Bar Press x 6 x 3 sets

4) Lat Pull downs 4 sets 10 reps

5) Three Board Close Grip x 3 x 3 sets (last set max reps)

Week 2

1) Bench Press 85 percent x 1 x 8 sets (rest 30 seconds between sets, last set as many reps as possible)

2) Isodynamic (at sticking point) x 3 sets

3) Two Board Cambered Bar Press x 6 x 3 sets

4) Lat Pull downs 4 sets 10 reps

5) Three Board Close Grip x 2 x 3 sets (last set max reps)

Week 3

1) Bench Press 90 percent x 1 x 6 sets (rest 30 seconds between sets, last set as many reps as possible)

2) Isodynamic (at sticking point) x 3 sets

3) Two Board Cambered Bar Press x 6 x 3 sets

4) Lat Pull downs 4 sets 10 reps

5) Three Board Close Grip x 1 x 3 sets (last set max reps)

Week 4
   ➢ Deload

Prison Yard Push Isometrics

Before California completely banned barbells in prisons in 1992, barbells topped out at 195 pounds. This was not enough weight for the stronger inmates. To increase resistance, cons would resist the barbell on both the way up and down, by having a lift partner act as extra resistance by pushing on the barbell. This ingenuity can help us free folks! Because we have the ability to handle much heavier weight on a negative

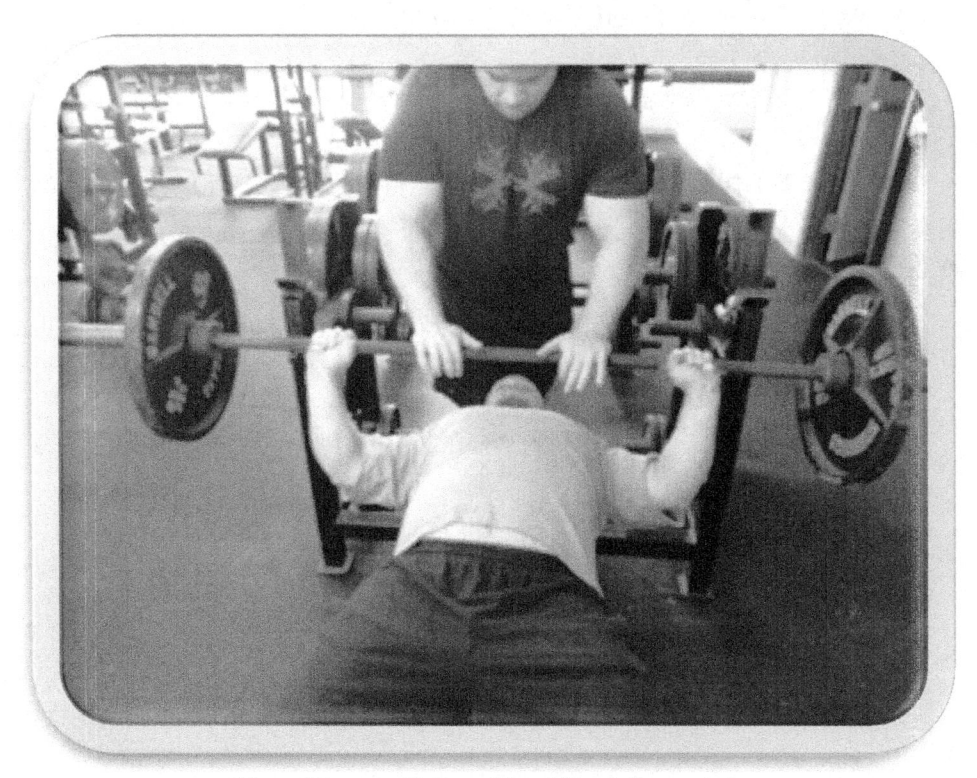

Ross Shreves Prison Yard Push Isometric

contraction, for our purposes a partner will resist on the way up. Load 70-85 percent of your one repetition max on the bar and perform the negative at normal speed. As you push the barbell back up, have a competent partner resist you with his hand at your sticking point, pushing with maximal force for 4-5 seconds. At that point, your partner will remove his hand, and you can forcefully push the weight to lockout.

There are a couple draw backs to this method, as it is nearly impossible for the same lifting partner to quantify how much resistance he is providing as you push up. If you train with different partners each session, quantification becomes an even more daunting task. You must push with maximal force. The other potential issue is a partner not capable of providing sufficient resistance, or an overzealous knuckle head that provides too much.

This method can help you overcome sticking points and build explosive power. The 70-85 percent is not gospel. Play around with the exact amount of weight that works best for you.

Isometric/CAT Contrast

Maximizing force production, eliminating sticking points, inhibiting force reduction safety mechanisms…the list goes on! This method can be used even if you are not working on a specific sticking point and just want to enhance explosive power.

Studies show the PAP effect is maximized between 1 and 7 minutes after a maximal isometric contraction. This method is done in the power rack. Put a bench in the power rack and set the pins at your sticking point. Lift an empty barbell from chest level to the pins. There is no reason to add weight because you are pushing against an immovable object. Once contact is made with the pins, push as hard as you can. Hold the maximal contraction for 5 seconds. Rest 1-7 minutes after the isometric, generally no more than 3 minutes is needed.

After your rest period, bench press a submaximal weight in CAT style. You will be more explosive. You can work up to 5 sticking points in one workout, up to 3 sets per point, but no more than 10 sets in one work is recommended. So if you work five points, only do 1-2 sets per point.

For general PAP training without addressing a specific sticking point, I recommend a bottom range point, mid-range point, and a top end point.

Let's take a look at practical application.

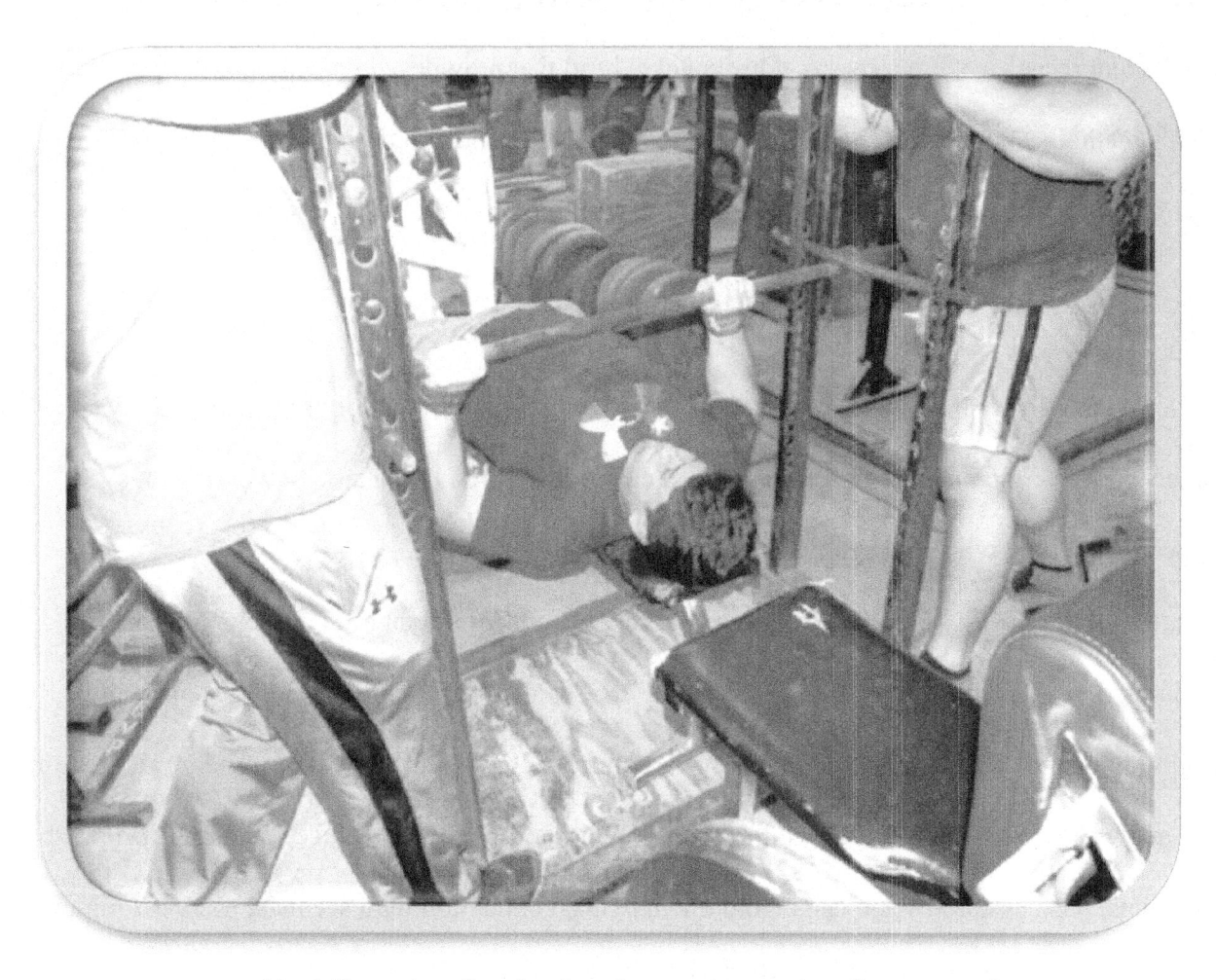

Noah Bryant performing bench press isometrics. Spotters make sure he does not lift the rack off the ground.

Isometric/CAT Contrast Routine

Week 1

1) Bench Press 90 percent x 2 reps

2) Bottom Level Isometric Rest 2 minutes CAT Bench Press rest 2 Minutes 75 percent x 3 reps x 2 sets

3) Mid-range Isometric Rest 2 minutes CAT Bench Press rest 2 Minutes 80 percent x 3 reps x 2 sets

4) Top-range Isometric Rest 2 minutes CAT Bench Press rest 2 Minutes 80 percent x 3 reps x 2 sets

5) Wide Grip Paused Bench Press-8 reps x 2 sets

6) Dicks Press-10,9,8,6 x 4 sets

7) Band Pushdowns-100 reps x 2 sets

Week 2

1) Bench Press 92.5 percent x 2 reps

2) Bottom Level Isometric Rest 2 minutes CAT Bench Press rest 2 Minutes 75 percent x 3 reps x 2 sets

3) Mid-range Isometric Rest 2 minutes CAT Bench Press rest 2 Minutes 80 percent x 3 reps x 2 sets

4) Top-range Isometric Rest 2 minutes CAT Bench Press rest 2 Minutes 85 percent x 3 reps x 2 sets

5) Wide Grip Paused Bench Press-7 reps x 2 sets

6) Dicks Press-8,7,7,6 x 4 sets

7) Band Pushdowns-100 reps x 2 sets

Week 3

1) Bench Press 95 percent x 1 rep x 3 sets

2) Bottom Level Isometric Rest 2 minutes CAT Bench Press rest 2 Minutes 75 percent 3 reps x 2 sets

3) Mid-range Isometric Rest 2 minutes CAT Bench Press rest 2 Minutes 82 percent x 3reps x 2 sets

4) Top-range Isometric Rest 2 minutes CAT Bench Press rest 2 Minutes 87.5 percent x 3 reps x 2 sets

5) Deep Dumbbell Paused Bench Press-8 reps x 2 sets

6) Rolling Dumbbell Triceps Extension -15 reps x 4 sets

7) Band Pushdowns-100 reps x 2 sets

Week 4 -- Deload

Isometrics paired with Compensatory Acceleration Training have worked wonders for both Vince Dizenzo and "Big Al" Davis.

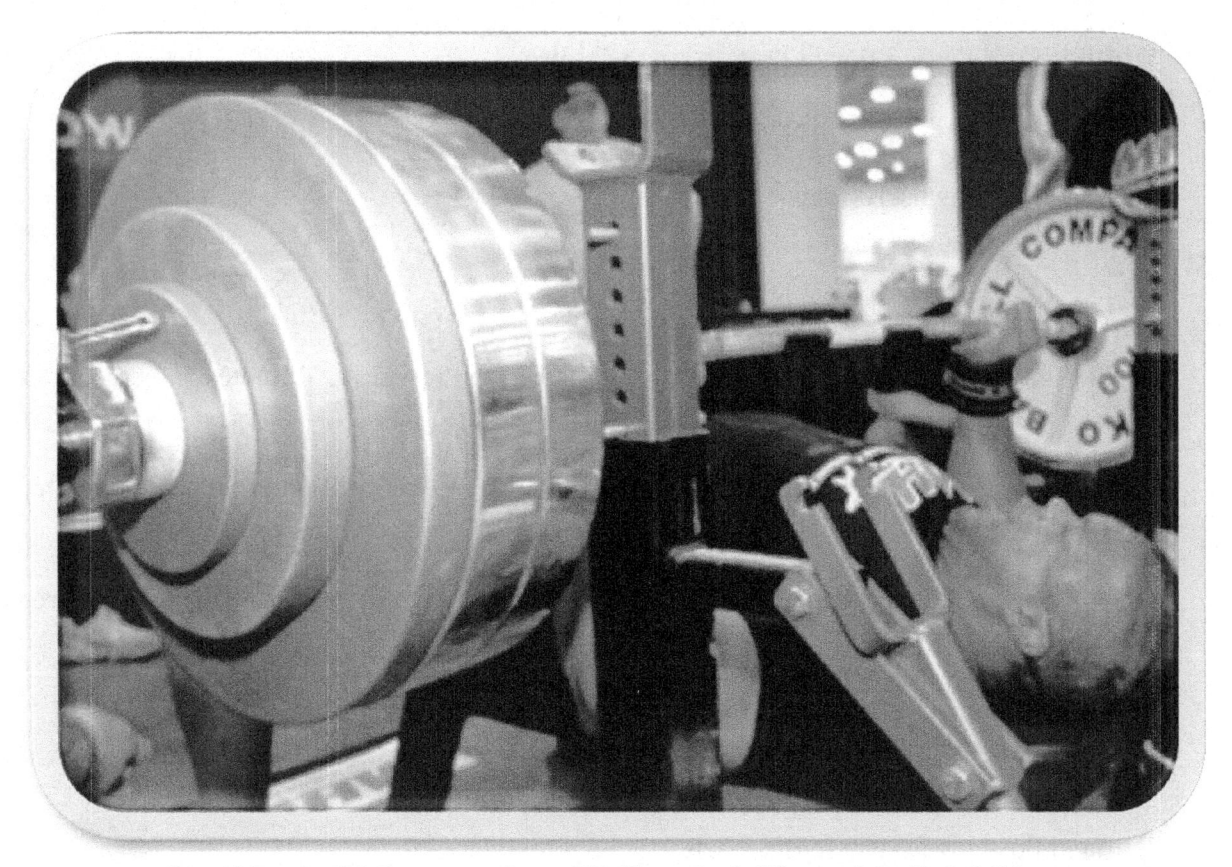

Big Al Davis 600 Opener at Seanzilla Katterles's Kings of the Bench Meet

Isometric Programming

Generally, these isometric variations are done in the last block preceding a meet. This helps get rid of any last minute sticking points and will push you over the edge to new personal records. They can be used in the off-season to address weaknesses.

The last three week block before a meet must be followed by a one week deload, then relative relaxation before a meet. Do not be afraid of losing the positive effects gained by this extreme method of developing limit strength. Residual training effects from limit strength training can offer a benefit up to a month after they have been discontinued according to Vladimir Issurin in his revolutionary book, Block Periodization.

Let's take a look at what science has to say.

Sticking Points-Cause and Effect

Is the occurrence of the sticking point a product of weakening potentiation (coinciding delayed muscle activation) or the result of a mechanically weak area in which muscles produce less force? This study set out to answer that question. A one-repetition max bench press was compared with isometrics (producing maximum force statically) throughout a dozen different regions of the bench press.

If lower force was produced at the sticking points isometrically compared to the other "stronger" points in the isometric bench press, this would validate that sticking points are a product of mechanically-weak positions where muscles produce less force. Twelve males with prior lifting experience ranging from 20-23 years maxed out in the bench press along with testing max force in 12 different regions of the bench press that they could produce isometrically.

In one repetition max tests, as well as isometric ones, mechanically weak areas were observed where less force could be produced. This study concluded sticking points are real and at certain points in the bench press people are able to produce less force, which results in a sticking point.

van den Tillaar, R., Saeterbakken, A., & Ettema, G. (2012). Is the occurrence of the sticking region the result of diminishing potentiation in bench press?. *Journal of Sports Sciences*, 30(6), 591-599

Practical Application

Some studies suggest sticking points are only a product of deceleration or too much time under tension. Deceleration is a result of decreased assistance of the stretch shortening cycle, coupled with reaching an area where force production significantly decreases. That's why I have outlined strategies that will strengthen specific sticking points.

Isometric and other supplementary movements outlined in the book will help strengthen specific mechanically weak areas of the bench press.

Final Thoughts

Bench pressing sticking points are like grass, and the isometric methods outlined are the lawn mower. Cut 'em down! You have been given the tools.

The Power of Positive Benching

Super slow negatives in the bench press were about as common in the 1980s and 1990s as the spandex that plagued the era.

Top bench pressers like Al Davis, Robert Wilkerson and Jeremy Hoorsntra are now crediting a large part of their bench press power to the dead bench.

Let's take a look at what science has to say.

Dead Bench Practically Applied

The dead bench should be performed for singles; even after you pause, almost half the elastic energy aids in the concentric. To achieve higher volume and lower intensity, use multiple singles followed by short rest intervals, instead of pumping out rep after rep. Proper progression is where many people fail in their strength programs. We can know science in and out, but if we don't understand the true art of progression, we will not progress. Some variables to increase intensity on the dead bench are shortening rest intervals between singles, adding more singles

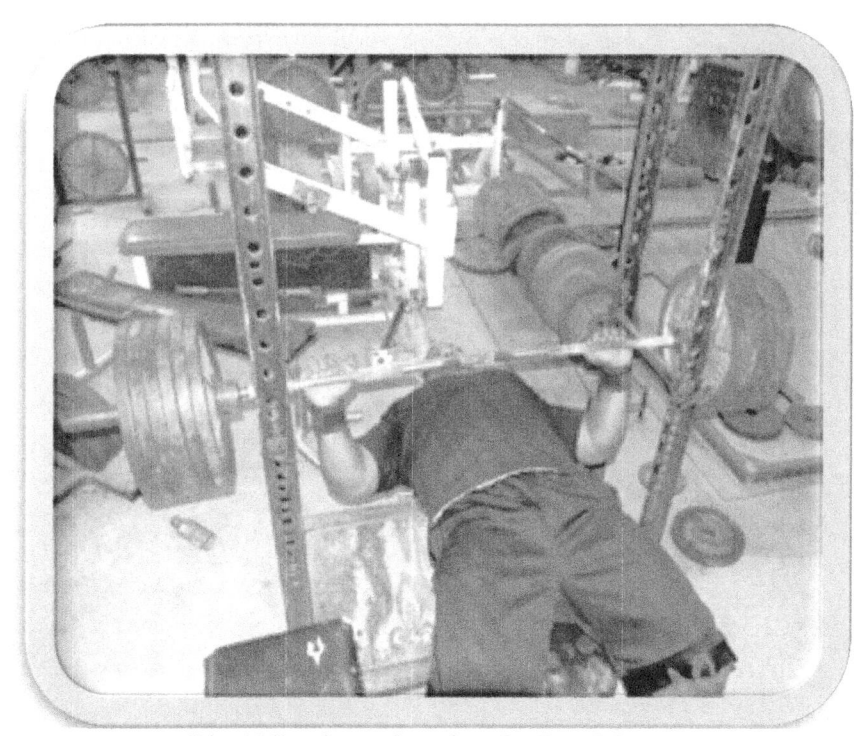

Big Al Davis performing the Dead Bench

to the same weight, and adding more weight. Then, you can also look at lengthening rest periods and decreasing the number of singles as the weight gets heavier. Looking only at bar weight is a good prescription to running yourself in the ground quickly.

Dead benches are not to be done in place of regular bench presses; the bench press is a reversible muscle action. The dead bench press is a concentric only muscle action. While this is a helpful accessory in building starting strength to get better at the bench press, you must bench press. How far off the chest? Variations can be from chest level to a couple inches off. Taller, longer-limbed lifters generally have more success placing the bar further off the chest because of the powerful stretch shortening cycle from the longer negative.

What should you be able to dead bench press? Approximately 85-95 percent of your one repetition max in the paused bench press. Although there is variation, long-limbed lifters generally do less. However, the long-armed bench presser has one distinct advantage - a longer eccentric and potentially, a more powerful stretch reflex to aid in pushing the weight back up.

If your dead bench press is the same as your regular bench press, you do not need to focus on this movement. Besides practicing technique in the competition bench press, focus on the enhancement of muscle elasticity specific to the bench press. This is done through bench plyometric variations, Compensatory Acceleration Training (CAT) bench presses, plyometrics, and, of course, technical practice.

How do you program the dead bench press? Again, this is a special preparatory exercise, not the core lift, so certainly some variation is allowed. Here is Option A, for someone running the dead bench press through the entirety of the 12 week training cycle:

Week	Exercise	Sets	Reps	Intensity Percentage	Rest Interval In Seconds
1	Dead Bench	8	1	60	30
2	Dead Bench	8	1	65	30
3	Dead Bench	6	1	70	45
4	Off	Off	Off	Off	Off
5	Dead Bench	5	1	75	90
6	Dead Bench	5	1	80	90
7	Dead Bench	4	1	70, 75, 80, 84	120
8	Off	Off	Off	Off	Off
9	Dead Bench	3	1	80, 83, 86	As Needed
10	Dead Bench	3	1	80, 84, 86	As Needed
11	Dead Bench	4	1	80, 85, 90	120
12	Off	Off	Off	Off	Off

That is an outline of how to use the dead bench press throughout the duration of a 12 week program. This does not have to be adhered to in stone. It is a guideline, but a successful one that has taken years of in-the-trenches experience to put together.

There are other approaches that can be taken to implement the dead bench press into your workout regimen. The first is the three week cyclical meso-cycle approach which should be used if you are constructing your strength building cycles in waves/blocks of three weeks, and you are rotating exercises you are using for accessory work on a three week basis. This approach can be used:

Week	Exercise	Sets	Reps	Intensity Percentage	Rest Interval In Seconds
1	Dead Bench	8	1	70	60
2	Dead Bench	4	1	75, 79, 82, 82	120
3	Dead Bench	?	1	80, 85, ??	As Needed

First, let's look at week one of this three week wave. If failure takes place before the duration of the singles are completed, initially, lower the weight by 5 percent and continue until you complete the prescribed number of sets/singles, which is four. In week two, if failure takes place, go back down to the last weight you completed and finish out the sets there. If you fail at your first set at 82 percent, go back down to 79 percent for the last two sets. Week three is your attempt to max. After finishing your sets of 80 and 85 percent, it is time to see what you are made of. Work up to a true max; do not be afraid of failure! However, you shouldn't strive for failure. If you hit a weight that you know is your true max, stop, move on and finish the rest of your workout.

The way to progress next time you cycle in this movement is progress from where you were previously. If you add five pounds to your week one, you have gotten better! If your last single week two is five pounds heavier, you have gotten better! If you beat your old max by five pounds week three, you have gotten better!

Legendary Strength Coach Charles Poliquin talks about the Japanese concept of Kaizen (改善?), which means "improvement," or "change for the better", and refers to the philosophy or practices that focus upon continuous improvement. With weights, this is should be very small increments. You can buy one-pound plates on Amazon for next to nothing. Don't blow your wad every time you dead bench.

If you want to rotate this exercise weekly, then the week three approach would be advisable, but one or two week rotations work. All of these percentages are based on your paused raw bench press max at the start of the 12 week training cycle.

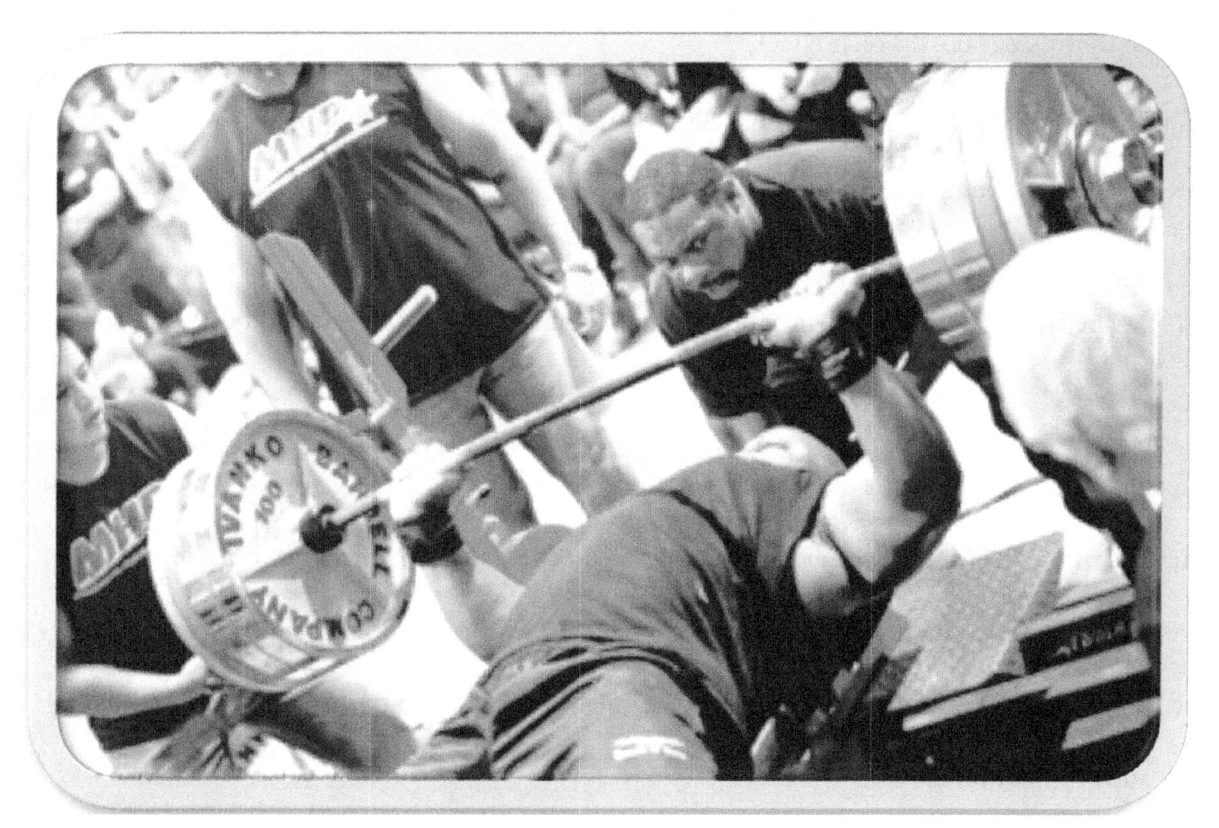

Big Al Davis 640 Pound Bench Press at Clash of the Titans Meet is Mesquite, Texas

Positive Verses Negatives for Strength Gains

The effects of training concentric (positive) with eccentric (negative) muscle actions on strength gains were examined. The study was performed on 42 subjects divided into three groups: the concentric experimental (CE), the eccentric experimental (EE) and a control (C).

The CE group trained with only concentric movements with 80 percent of their one repetition max in the bench press and bicep curl. The EE group trained with only eccentric movements but used 120 percent of their maxes in the same lifts.

Both of the groups performed three sets of 10-12 repetitions for eight weeks of both movements. The control group did not train at all. Both groups made significant increases in muscle strength. The CE group, however, did significantly outperform the EE group on the bicep curl and results were similar on the bench press.

This study was performed on novices.

The study concluded: Beginners should perform concentric muscle actions in the first eight weeks of weight training in order to gain strength at an accelerated pace.

De Carvalho Nogueira, A., De Souza Vale, R., Colado, J., Tella, V., Garcia-Masso, X., & Dantas, E. (2011). The effects of muscle actions upon strength gains. *Human Movement*, 12(4), 331-336.

Practical Applications

Eccentric muscle actions are associated with increased swelling and muscle damage, and greater amounts of the delayed onset muscle soreness when compared to concentric muscle actions. If strength gains were similar in both groups, concentric actions would be superior because they used 40 percent less weight and you can potentially perform them more frequently, something this study did not investigate.

Another interesting note in this study is velocity of movement was controlled; subjects were required to take three seconds on a concentric and three seconds on a negative. This is a huge red flag! The primary objective of eccentric emphasis training is to draw out the eccentric. The primary objective of a "dead movement" or concentric only is to develop starting strength. This is done by moving the weight as explosively as possible from start to finish. A force controlled concentric tempo will compromise the benefits of a dead movement. In spite of this error in design, concentric actions proved to yield greater gains! Imagine what happens when you do them right.

Dead movements (concentrics) build starting strength (how quickly you can develop tension in a muscle), acceleration strength, explosive strength, superior neural adaptations with faster recovery, and less muscle hypertrophy, an extremely important factor for a powerlifter looking to remain within a weight class.

The bench press is a reversible muscle action, meaning it has an eccentric and a concentric muscle. This is why most of your training should consist of reversible muscle action bench pressing. Concentric only dead benches play an important role in developing explosive power. Even with a 1/3 reduction in weight used, they yielded superior results to negatives, when not executed correctly.

Just think of the results performing dead benches with maximum force as explosively as possible.

Final Thoughts

Equipped bench pressers are notorious for allocating training effort toward lockout strength. For the raw bench presser starting strength is the name of the game. Anecdotes of top bench pressers confirm the effectiveness of dead bench presses. You now know the how and the why. Bring your bench press alive with the dead bench!

Explosive Bench Pressing: Plyometrics and Throws

In a nut shell, The Principle of Specificity conveys that to become better at a particular exercise or skill, you must perform that exercise or skill. To be a good bench presser, you must bench press. Hence, CAT bench press is the obvious choice for building an explosive bench press. Let's look at some alternative methods, shall we?

Plyometrics and bench press specific throws can aid your explosive pressing quest and even offer some benefits CAT does not.

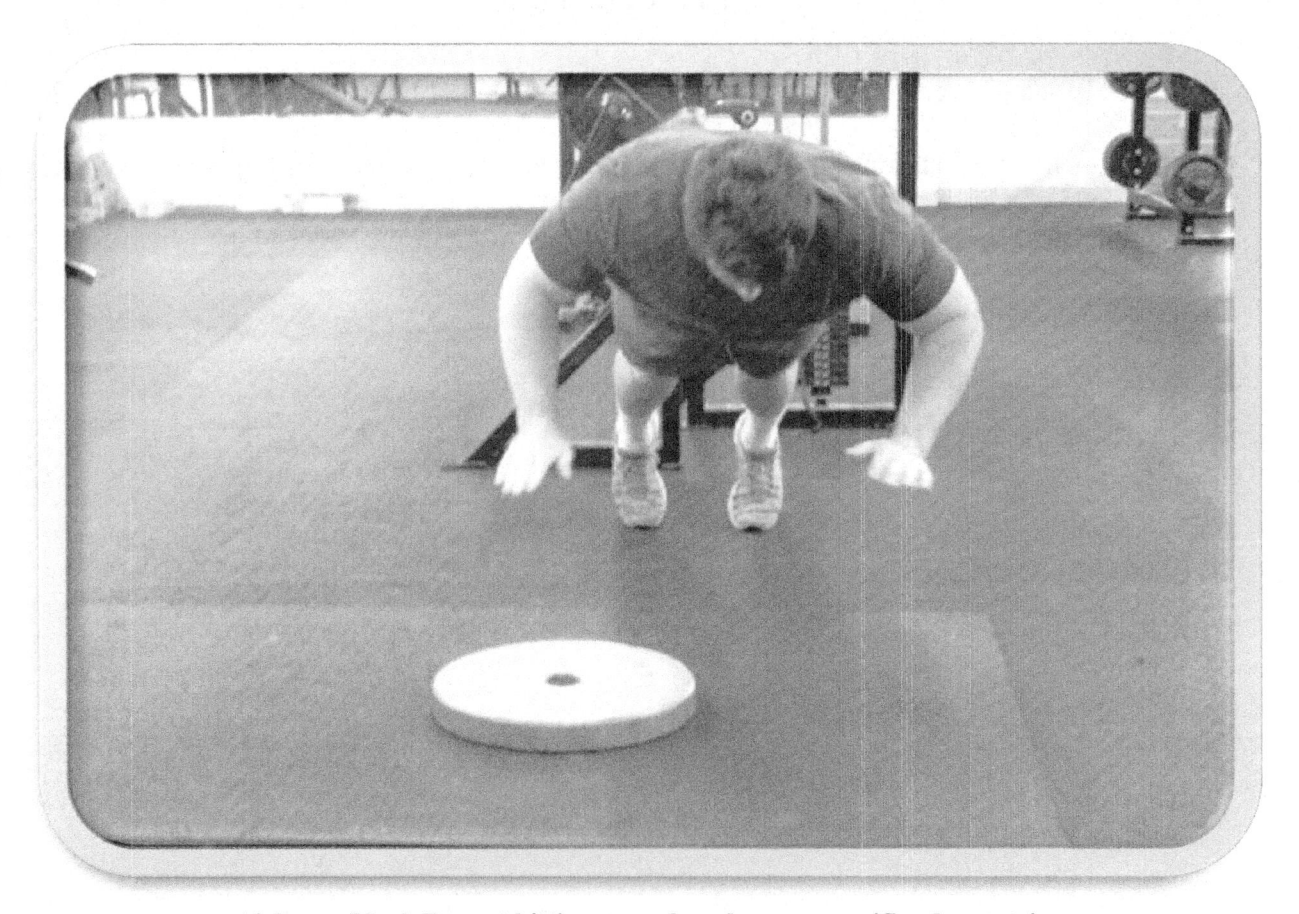

Airborne Noah Bryant hitting some bench press specific plyometrics

Bench Press: Phase 1, 2, & 3

In the bench press, as you push the barbell off your chest to lockout, I divide the upward movement into three phases.

> Phase 1 - *Initial Acceleration Phase* - the weight is pushed from a paused position on the chest to maximum speed.
>
> Phase 2 - *Constant Speed Phase* - the objective is to maintain the speed off the chest.
>
> Phase 3 - *Deceleration Phase* - the weight slows toward lockout to avoid hyperextension of the joint. This sounds like a blessing but it's a bench pressing curse, this safety mechanism acts way too early to the untrained bench presser.

Thank goodness for plyos and throws to combat this force inhibiting mechanism!

Bench Press and Sprinting

In the 100-meter dash after the first 45-55 meters, or five to six seconds, you reach maximum velocity. Your objective becomes maintaining maximum speed can as long as possible, usually three seconds. This is coined speed endurance.

Turning Off Inhibitory Mechanisms

The same principles that apply to the 100-meter dash apply to the bench press. In sprinting, the deceleration phase sets in because of a lack of speed endurance. In the bench press, speed endurance is not the issue; it's your body prematurely offering protection.

The triceps are the prime mover in the bench press lockout. The biceps serve as the antithesis to a forceful bench press lockout in the name of safety. CAT bench pressing has limits in developing maximum force through the entire range of motion. Bands and chains, discussed later in the text, have been helpful in overcoming this limiting factor, because lifters are forced to push with more force as they lockout a bench press.

You can defy the limitations imposed by lockout by pushing yourself off the ground, airborne with bench press specific plyometrics or throwing the bar beyond lock out with bench press specific throws.

Not only will this bring long-term explosive strength gains, this can immediately enhance more ability to bench more.

Let's take a look at practical application.

Bench Press Specific Plyometrics

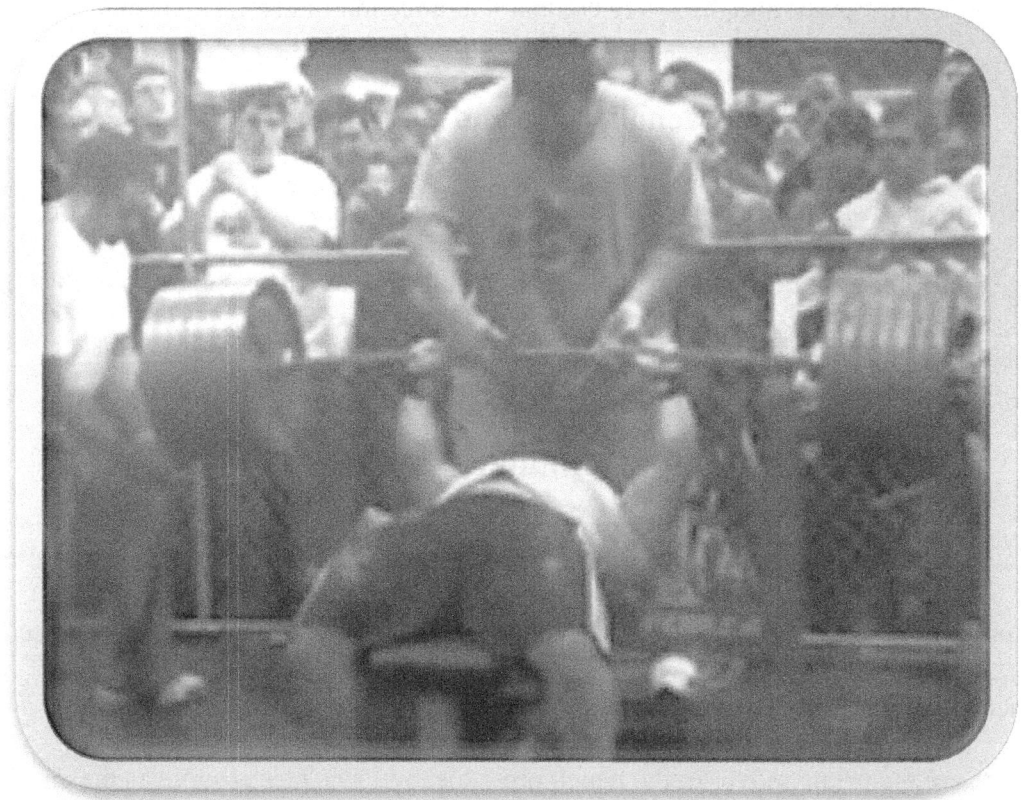

Jeremy Hoornstra Attempting 675 pounds in an exhibition with the late Nick Winters 650 pound raw bench presser spotting.

Here are some of my favorite bench press plyometrics:

- Depth Jump Push-up (Long Response): Start by lying in a push-up position with your hands on top of a stable surface, like a four inch box. For the downward phase, move your hands from the top of the surface down to the floor, keeping your hands slightly wider than your shoulders. Allow your chest to come about an inch off the box. For the upward phase, push up as fast and as high off the ground as possible, and land in the starting position, and then repeat. Do this for 2-4 sets of 3-6 reps.

- Depth Jump Push-up (Short Response): Same starting position as the long response depth jump push-up. Downward phase is again the same as the long response depth jump. Immediately, when the hands hit the ground, be ready to come back to lockout on top of the box. For the upward phase, push up as fast and high off the ground as high as possible and land in the starting position, then repeat. Do this for 2-4 sets of 3-6 reps.

- Explosive Push-ups: Start by lying in a push-up position with one hand on a 3-4 inch surface and the other hand on the floor. For hand spacing, try and replicate your competition bench press grip or the grip you will use for your max, we are after transfer of training. Come down until your chest touches the box. For the upward phase, explode in the air as high as possible. Land on the box. Repeat. Do this for 2-4 sets of 3-6 reps.

- Upper Body Box Jumps-There should be a box or bench of appropriate height for your ability (between 3 and 16 inches) placed next to each other. Assume a push-up position between the two boxes (your shoulder width will determine the distance between the boxes. You should have approximately 2-4 inches of free space on either side).

Explosively thrust your upper body upward and land with your hands on each box. "Step" down easily before your next repetition. Don't try and just get up to the box, get maximum height each jump. Perform this for singles, 3-12 will suffice.

- Medicine Ball Drops Most medicine ball drills can be done not by catching the ball, rather by repelling it. Lie on the ground. Have a partner stand above you and throw the ball toward your hands with your arms extended and don't catch the ball! Rather, cradle it and push it back up as forcefully as possible. The idea is to resist the eccentric contraction and push the ball back up as high as possible as fast as possible. Think of the ball as being red-hot and one you want to spend as little time in contact with as possible. Do this for 3-6 repetitions; the idea is to build explosive power, not endurance.

Recently, another strategy that I have used is Smith machine bench throws, using 10-20 percent of a client's bench press max. Throw the weight as high as possible; triples work well for 3-6 sets. This improves elasticity efficiency. Even after a one-second pause, nearly half of elastic energy is still present! Most meets won't make you pause that long.

Remember, strength is primarily a function of the nervous system. By literally throwing the weights, the neural factors that want to keep you down can be trained to be suppressed with this method.

Let's take a look at what science has to say.

Explosive Movements Activate Limit Strength in the Bench Press

Some have theorized that explosive-force movements prior to heavy bench presses would equate to a higher one repetition max (1RM). Let's take a look by turning to our guiding light, science.

Twelve male college athletes with previous strength training and bench press experience participated in three testing sessions divided by minimally five days of rest. Throughout all testing sessions, the one repetition max was measured on the bench press. Subjects first performed a general warm-up, followed by a specific warm-up comprised of submaximal weights, each set increased load on the bench press exercise prior to attempting a one rep bench max. Through the first testing trial, the subjects attempted a sequence of one repetition max efforts with increasing loads before determining their one repetition max. Throughout the second and third testing trials, subjects executed in a randomized order either two plyometric push-ups or two medicine-ball (3 to 5 kg) chest passes 30 seconds prior to attempting a one repetition max. The results echo some potential benefits for the raw bench press aficionado: one repetition max bench press strength was considerably greater after performing plyometric push-ups or chest passes, contrasted with the initial trial. This study concluded that low-volume, explosive-force upper body movements completed 30 seconds prior to a one repetition max could potentially increase the bench press max in trained subjects. This would be via the PAP effect. The PAP effect is believed to induce factors that help muscles produce more force immediately via chemical, neural, and mechanical changes in muscle tissue.

This particular study showed one repetition max bench press strength was considerably better after PAP plyometric push-ups by 4 percent or PAP medicine ball chest passes by 2.5 percent, in contrast with the first pilot, which was a more traditional warm-up.

Wilcox, J., Larson, R., Brochu, K. M., & Faigenbaum, A. D. (2006). Acute Explosive-Force Movements Enhance Bench-Press Performance in Athletic Men. *International Journal of Sports Physiology & Performance*, **1(3), 261-269.**

Practical Application

We must conclude that a performance of an explosive movement before a one repetition max excites the central nervous system and subsequently allows the athlete to lift more weight. Explosive-force movements may be responsible for motor neuron excitability and reflex potentiation, resulting in a higher one repetition max. In other words, your central nervous system recruits more help to get the job done faster, so you can lift more weight. Simply, when it comes to lifting maximum weights, the more help the better.

The conclusion of other studies is that trained athletes benefit more from PAP than beginners. All subjects in this study were athletes involved in sports that require the ability to produce large amounts of high force and explosive power. Researchers concluded that explosive movements can enhance neural stimulation to a point that will significantly increase an athlete's one repetition max in the bench press.

In this study, subjects' one repetition max in the bench press improved about 2.5 percent after PAP protocols as equated with a customary testing procedure deprived of PAP.

When people ask me when to perform plyometric push-ups, a standard answer is: before a workout, so long as you have a sufficient work capacity. When asked why, I would simply respond that I'd feel stronger and more explosive. Well, this study confirmed using plyometric push-ups or medicine ball throws before lifting maximal weight. The object is to perform these movements as explosively as possible for low repetitions, nowhere near the level of fatigue, and you will be able to lift more weight.

Just think, a 2.5 percent increase on a 600-pound bench press is 12.5 pounds!! That's huge. This information used wisely can help propel you to the next level, but if it is abused, it can help you perform a pseudo pre-exhaust technique.

Weight Releasers Increase Power

If you lower additional weight on the negative of the bench press, can you push more up on the positive phase? This study examined that.

Eight subjects with some weight training experience lifted maximal attempts in the bench press using detaching hooks (weight releasers) lowering 105 percent of their bench press one repetition maximum (1-RM) and lifting back up their max. The weight releasers permitted additional weight on the bar and released from the barbell at the bottom of the bench press, reducing the weight subjects had to push back up.

After establishing a bench press max, the subjects tried to increase their max by using a heavier eccentric load with additional weight releasers. All eight increased their bench presses by 5 to 15 pounds.

A heavier negative increased the subjects' bench press maxes by an average of 8 percent. Researchers stated, "This phenomenon was a result of the enhancement of stretch-shortening cycle performance by the increased eccentric load. Athletes who are interested in developing one repetition max strength in the bench press may benefit from the use of additional eccentric loading."

Doan, B. K., Newton, R. U., Marsit, J. L., Triplett-McBride, N. N., Koziris, L. P., Fry, A. C., & Kraemer, W. J. (2002). Effects of increased eccentric loading on bench press one repetition max. *Journal of Strength & Conditioning Research* **(Allen Press Publishing Services Inc.), 16(1), 9-13.**

Practical Application

Weight releasers are a great tool to help build a big bench! Generally, the more advanced the lifter, the more pronounced the effect with increased eccentric loading. It is amazing this effect was so powerful in subjects "with some lifting experience." Weight releasers can be used by as much as 15-20 percent above your one repetition max. The idea is not to use such a heavy weight that you have trouble controlling it. If the weight is too heavy, you will not benefit from the elastic-like properties of the stretch reflex. Your body will seek to protect you, not to lift more.

To build power in the bench press, generally, there is no need to lower greater than 10 percent over your one repetition max. Use weight releasers wisely. Keep in mind eccentric overloads cause a greater delayed onset of muscle soreness (DOMS) and take much longer to recover. Weight releasers are a supplement for the traditional bench press, not a substitute. Used correctly, this tool can help enhance rate of force production, provide an overload of handling supramaximal weight and enhance limit strength.

Wearing Off of Stretch Reflex Causes Sticking Point

This study analyzed the bench press of 10 elite powerlifters using three-dimension cinematography and surface electromyography. Athletes bench pressed 80 percent of their 1 RM, a 1 RM, and a failed supramaximal attempt.

Through data analysis, the study concluded: The sticking point was not caused by an increase in weight about the shoulder or elbow joints or by decreased muscle activation. Researchers concluded a possible cause of the force-reduced transition phase between a strain energy-assisted acceleration phase and a mechanically advantageous maximum strength region is postulated. In other words, after the energy you stored on the negative is done helping you on the way up, the weight slows, and you stick!

Elliott, B. C., Wilson, G. J., & Kerr, G. K. (1989). A biomechanical analysis of the sticking region in the bench press. *Medicine & Science in Sports & Exercise,* **21(4), 450-462.**

Practical Application

Most powerlifting meets will have less than a one second pause, so an efficient stretch shortening cycle is a must. This can be developed with CAT bench presses, bench press with bands, bench presses with chains and bench press specific plyometrics.

Final Thoughts

Sticking points do not exist if you by-pass them with enough bar speed. Forcing limiting factors can be "forced" to get lost with modalities outlined in this chapter. Become a more explosive bench presser, become a stronger bench presser.

Sound Science or Bro Science?

Some traditional training methods are blindly accepted by gym-goers as Gospel.

Let's take a look at what science has to say.

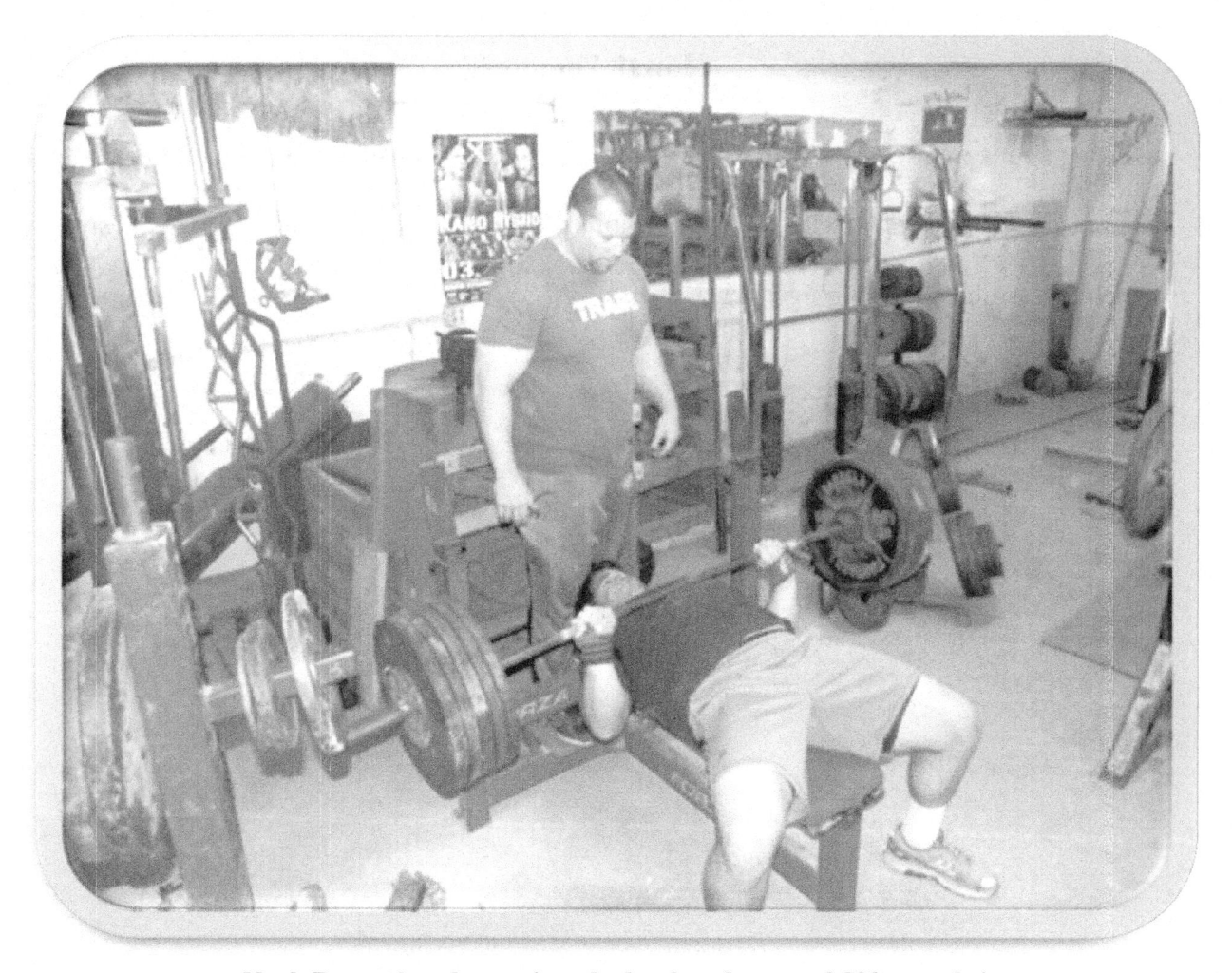

Noah Bryant bench pressing - he has bench pressed 500 pounds in competition. Here Noah Bench presses 505 at Metroflex Gym.

Muscle Activation: Fat Bar verses Standard Bar

Many believe muscle activation is greater when using a fat bar (two inch diameter) compared to a standard bar (1.1 inch diameter.) This was examined when subjects performed the bench press under both conditions at various spots isometrically.

The researchers concluded:

"Our data does not support the hypothesis that bar diameter influences performance during an isometric bench press exercise. Our data does not support the use of a fat bar for increasing neuromuscular activation"

Fioranelli, D., Lee, C. (2008) The influence of bar diameter on neuromuscular strength and activation: Inferences from an isometric unilateral bench press. *Journal of Strength & Conditioning Research (Lippincott Williams & Wilkins), 22(3), 661-666.*

Practical Application

Like unstable surfaces, fat bars do not increase muscle activation. Some lifters report less joint pain while training with fat bars; while this may be true, the benefits don't go beyond that to neuromuscular activation. A majority of your training needs to take place how you compete, with an Olympic bar.

Static Stretching and the Bench Press

The one repetition bench press max of 20 Jiu-Jitsu athletes was assessed in this study. Maxes

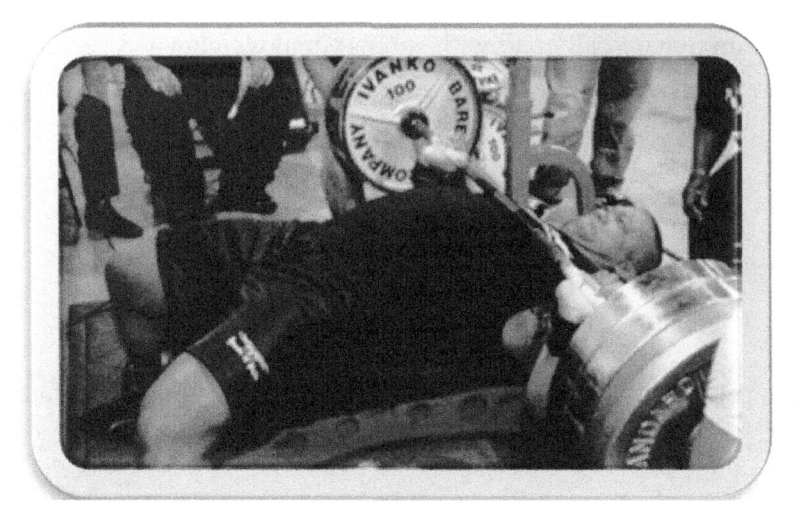

Big Al Davis getting ready to blast a 635 pound raw bench

were tested with and without performing static stretching prior to testing. The static stretching consisted of three separate static stretching exercises performed for three sets held for 20 seconds each. Stretches were performed on the primary bench press muscles.

After subjects stretched, their one repetitions maxes averaged 8.75 percent lower than without the stretching protocol.

Costa, E., dos Santos, C., Prestes, J., da Silva, J., & Knackfuss, M. (2009). Acute effect of static stretching on the strength performance of jiu-jitsu athletes in horizontal bench press. *Fitness & Performance Journal* **(Online Edition), 8(3), 212-217.**

Practical Application

When I first started training raw bench press phenomenon Al Davis, he told me that he always had his best meets when he didn't have enough time to warm-up. His best workouts fell on days he arrived at the gym and didn't have time to warm up. A light bulb went off in my head! I asked if he still warmed up with light weights, and he said yes. The difference was he didn't have time to stretch. Al's best workouts resulted from being rushed because he did not static stretch beforehand.

If you want to lift maximal weights, don't static stretch before hand, as a plethora of studies have confirmed. You will feel "loose" and activate the golgi tendon organ (mechanism that inhibits force production). You should warm-up dynamically and with submaximal weights before bench pressing. Save static stretching for post workout.

Final Thoughts

What initially appears to be sound science, on further investigation, might "bro science." Tradition by no means equals sound science. Accept nothing in the strength world on blind faith.

Partials for Raw Bench Pressers

Enough speed off the chest can help you chop down any sticking point in your path. Partials are not the name of the game like many well-meaning, equipped lifters will have you believe, but they certainly can find a home in the regimen of the raw powerlifter!

Here are some strategies I have used with partial movements:

Board Presses

Board presses are the bread and butter exercise for many top equipped lifters. Board presses potentially offer a multitude of benefits to the raw powerlifter. Great overload can take place because of the above maximal poundages that can be used on board presses. Board presses also can help build power in the range where the power built from dead stop benches and

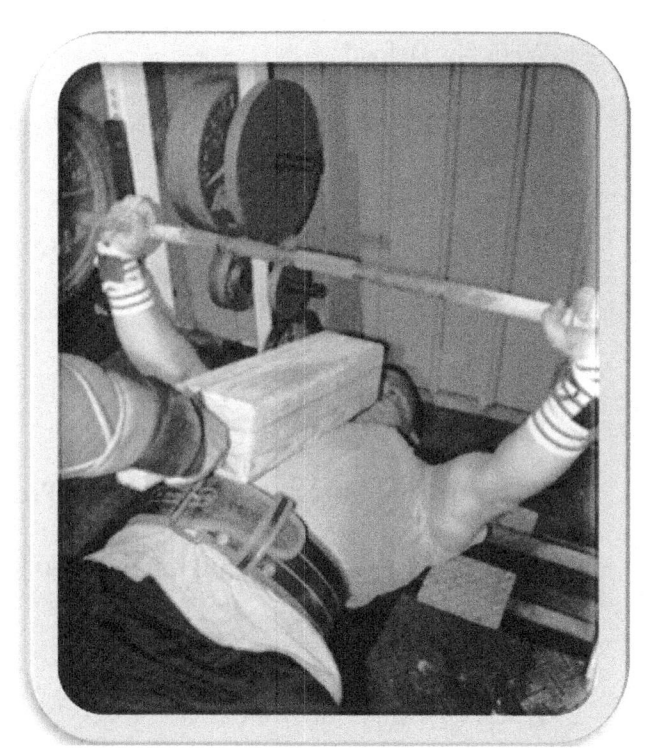

Three Board Press training at the EliteFTS Compound

plyometrics wears off. Furthermore, they can be used to work the bench press lockout or even directly target sticking points. Board presses even allow guys with bad shoulders to keep on pressing! I have had powerlifting clients with poor shoulder and pec health train primarily with boards and go on to bench press very successfully in raw power meets. This is not advisable unless working around an injury, but it certainly beats the alternative of early retirement. Here is what a potential training cycle looks like for someone with poor shoulder health who can only bench press very infrequently.

12 Week Full ROM Injury: Board Press Cycle

Week 1 - Board Bench Press

Week 2 - Full Range of Motion Bench Press

Week 3 - Board Press

Week 4 - Deload

Week 5 - Full Range of Motion Bench Press

Week 6 - Two Board Bench Press

Week 7 - Reverse Band 1 Board Press

Week 8 - Deload

Week 9 - Two Board Press

Week 10 - Full Range of motion Bench Press

Week 11 - Reverse Band full range of motion bench Press

Week 12 - Deload

Week 13 - Max out or meet

Board Press Transference

Going past two boards will really decrease transference from the full range of motion bench press. Three and four board presses can be used to attack the midrange point of the bench press, and five and six board presses to attack the lockout. This will, of course, depend on the individual leverage of the lifter and structural weaknesses. Guys with alligator arms generally don't need high board work. Guys over six feet with knuckles that drag on the floor generally can derive benefit from higher board work.

Progressive Distance Training

Boards do provide a sufficient overload to targeted portions of the bench press. The potential down fall is the lack of transition phases. At some point, there will be a major change in mechanical advantage. When it is worsened, this is overcome by successfully made transitions through the movement. One archaic method of training in the power rack is progressive distance training. This involves lifting a weight off the pins in the power rack for a partial range of motion but instead of adding weight to the bar progressively, lower the pins in the rack. At first this method will work very well, but likely, you will run into a major sticking point. The bar will stop moving. Lifters have used this method more successfully with the squat and deadlift. This happens simply because the transition phases are eliminated, so the sticking point is much more pronounced.

If you want to experiment with progressive distance training, I suggest doing so with boards. Make each board approximately one quarter inch. This way you get an eccentric and concentric phase like a regular bench press.

For dead movements or concentric only movements, the rack is your choice. For reversible muscle action (both a negative and positive), boards, rack press seven days a week and twice on Sunday. The difference is more pronounced than you might think. In the bottom position of a rack press, the energy of the weight is transferred into the rack, dissipating into the ground. This is not a factor for the dead bench because all that matters is pushing the weight up in a bottom up fashion, not the redirection of force from a negative to a positive. Technique reinforcement is more likely with board presses because board presses allow less room for error, forcing you to stay tight. If you lose tightness on a rack press, the rack can absorb the weight, which is not the case with board presses.

Additionally, board presses have one point of contact with the bar (center of the chest) and rack presses have two points of contact, the metal pins of the rack. The groove will feel much more "real," like your raw bench pressing technique, when board pressing.

There is no secret formula to the implementation of board presses. If you are weak off the bottom, low boards are the order. If you stick in the mid-range, that's where work needs to be done, and if you struggle toward the top end, that's where attention needs to be paid. Blend board pressing off of different heights with CAT training, and sticking points will be on the ash heap of your lifting history!

Board presses can be used for limit strength work at or above your one repetition max, repetition work, burnouts or even drop sets. Board presses are not just for shirted benchers anymore!

Rack Lockout Overloads

Rack lockouts don't generally offer the transfer of training one might expect. When you miss a weight at lockout, generally, you are out of position, or there is some sort of technical break down. This movement should not be dismissed.

Simply put a flat bench inside a squat rack and set the bar across the pins where you will only have to move the barbell two to four inches. This is a great chance to use supramaximal weights. By using these weights you will build some lockout strength, but more importantly, handle heavy weights. When you get to a meet and you are attempting to lift a personal record, this unchartered territory will not be such a shock. Because of the heavy weights used in training, be mindful when training heavy partials. It is not difficult to over train. Heavy partials can be used three weeks in a row, and then a cessation is needed.

Let's take a look at what science has to say.

Partial Overload Training

After testing partial range of motion bench presses in one session, four days later subjects were able to increase their one repetition and five repetition maxes significantly by 4.8 percent and 4.1 percent. Subjects were experienced bodybuilders and powerlifters who had trained exclusively with full range of motion bench presses.

This study showed that strength differences can occur rapidly after one session with exposure to partial ROM exercises.

Mookerjee, S. S., & Ratamess, N. N. (1999). Comparison of strength differences and joint action durations between full and partial range-of-motion bench press exercise. *Journal of Strength & Conditioning Research* **(Allen Press Publishing Services Inc.), 13(1), 76-81.**

Practical Application

Dynamic partial range of motion (partial ROM) training is an advanced strength-training technique used by many shirted bench pressers. Raw lifters are catching on! Zatsiorsky has described the accentuation principle, in other words to train in the range of motion where the highest amounts of force are produced.

By training partials with supramaximal weights the CNS will become accustomed to heavy weights, neural inhibitions will decline. The powerlifter can train partial range of motion with board presses and pin presses. Partials do eliminate transitional phases within the bench presses. This can be circumvented with adding chains or elastic band resistance to the barbell while performing a full range of motion bench press.

The researchers concluded "Individuals who train exclusively in a full ROM may fail to optimally train in the area of the ROM where maximal force development occurs." This is certainly true, but full range of motion with bands and chains can provide the overload benefit of partials, without eliminating transition phases. Remember, bench press is your bread and butter, but man cannot live off of bench press alone!

Final Thoughts

Partials for raw bench pressers can be an important piece of the pie. The key is to remember partials are a supplement to full range of motion work not a substitute. Used correctly, partials can provide a boost to the raw bench press.

Bands and Chains for the Raw Bench Presser

Bands and chains provide a great overload and complement strength curve of bench press. Bands speed up the eccentric portion of the movement. Chains bridge the gap between bands and straight weight. These are a great way to build lockout strength with full range of motion and transitions.

The issue with partials that overload specific ranges of motion is simply the lack of transitional phases that all real core lifts have. The solution that gives the most economical response to this question is the implementation of bands and chains. Bands and chains allow you to still perform the full range of motion. Transitional phases are not eliminated, but sufficient overload is achieved because as leverage improves, resistance increases.

Generally, for raw powerlifters and strongmen, I recommend 10-25 percent additional bands or chains to the barbell weight. For a barbell loaded with 400 pounds, this would be an additional 40 to 100 pounds of accommodated resistance. This is a guideline and certainly not a rule. There is a time and a

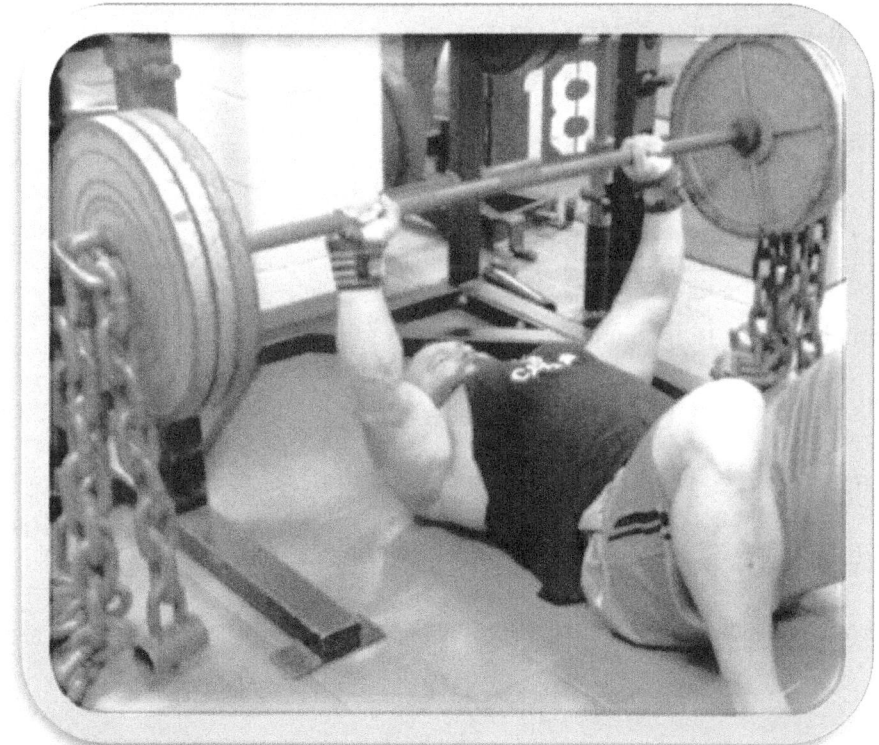

BJ Whitehead performing floor presses with additional chain resistance

place for specific overloads. The issue would be using literally two to three times the bar weight with additional bands or chains, like many equipped lifters do.

Let's take a look at what science has to say.

Bands Enhance Bench Press Strength and Power

Strength and power adaptations of combined elastic band and barbell training with traditional barbell-only training were examined. Forty-four young men, 19-21 years old with serious strength training backgrounds, tested maxes before and after seven weeks of training. One group performed back squats and bench presses with barbell and weights only, the other group combined barbell and weights with additional elastic bands. The band group nearly tripled gains on the squat over the traditional group and doubled gains in the bench press. The band group had significant improvement on power development.

Anderson, C. E., Sforzo, G. A., & Sigg, J. A. (2008). The effects of combining elastic and free weight resistance on strength and power athletes. *Journal of Strength & Conditioning Research* **(Lippincott Williams & Wilkins), 22(2), 567-574.**

Practical Applications

Numerous studies show the positive effects of bands on bench press strength and power. Training with bands allows overload throughout the entire range of motion. For lifters with shoulder injuries that want to keep on pressing, opt for reverse band bench presses. Regular bench presses are your core movement, band bench

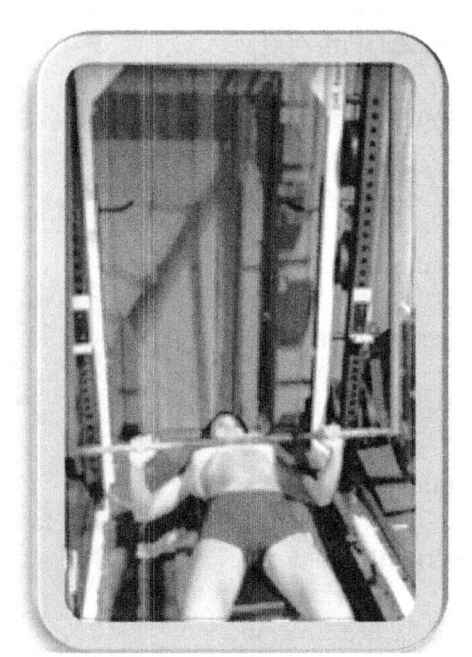

Reverse Band Bench Presses at the EliteFTS Compound

presses are a helpful adjunct that can help take your pressing strength and power to the next level.

Train with Chains and Bench More

With all this talk about chains, let's look to science. This study compared a bench press strength training regimen with chains added to the barbell to traditional training for the bench press with no additional chain weight.

Women collegiate athletes in volleyball and basketball were the subjects for this study which spanned over 16 bench press sessions. Groups were divided into a traditional or a chain training group. The traditional group bench pressed with a barbell and weights with no added variable resistance, and the chain group trained with 5 percent additional chains added to the barbell. Analysis showed a significant increase in the one repetition max for both groups over 16 sessions, but the chain group improved by nearly six percent more on average.

Burnham, T. R., Ruud, J. D., & McGowan, R. (2010). Bench press training program with attached chains for female volleyball and basketball athletes. *Perceptual & Motor Skills*, 110(1), 61-68.

Practical Application

Chains are generally thought of as a tool for advanced powerlifters. This study raises some questions. Female collegiate basketball and volleyball players are not thought of as having extreme physical prowess in the bench press, but even so, they benefited from additional chain resistance. Some work outs should use chains, other should not. Yet, all work outs for all work sets included chains. This is more than most coaches would suggest, so how did the athletes improve?

Athletes improved because as you forcefully push the bar to completion on the bench press, your biceps serve as the antagonist to your triceps; in other words, biceps slow down bar speed so you don't hyperextend your elbows.

The problem is this built-in safety mechanism acts way too quickly!! Chains get heavier and heavier as you approach lockout, so you produce higher amounts of force longer. Because of built-in safety mechanisms like the antagonist muscle and Golgi Tendon Organ (GTO), chains allow you to train to somewhat inhibit these force reducing actions because you have to push harder and longer, a result of the variable resistance of the chains.

Sticking points result where athletes are able to produce less force, so athletes need to push the barbell as quickly as possible with as much force as possible to keep it moving. Chains amplify this effect. You have no choice but to hit the gas. If you lay on the cruise control, the lift will fail. For beginners, this teaches Compensatory Acceleration Training!

Bench Press with Chains: Strength Gains, Shoulder Pain and Muscle Soreness

This study, performed on collegiate baseball players with resistance training experience, set out to compare the training effects on highly skilled athletes with a bench press regimen consisting of the traditional bench press (no additional chain weight) compared to a regimen that consisted of bench pressing with additional chain weight.

Researchers compared strength gains, shoulder pain, and muscle soreness induced by both regimens.

One repetition max (1-RM) values were assessed for both the traditional and chain program prior to the commencement of the program. The athletes were tested for a second time at the culmination of the nine-week training period to determine the level of strength gains achieved.

Subjects additionally were measured on 15 different occasions for muscle soreness and shoulder pain.

A linear progression periodization scheme was utilized, bench pressing heavy one day a week and light during the second session. Researchers attempted to keep training intensity and volume for both groups equal.

The results were interesting!

From the standpoint of shoulder pain, subjects bench pressing with chains experienced less than subjects using the traditional mode.

Strength gains for both groups were virtually identical, calling into the question the principle of specificity.

At the end of the study, the chain bench press group experienced a greater amount of muscle soreness than the traditional bench press group.

Chained Superiority? (2009). *Journal of Pure Power*, 4(2), 20-23.

Practical Application

To get better at the bench press, you have to bench press; of course, to say otherwise would contradict the principle of specificity. This study questions that! But, before we throw out everything we have ever known, let's look at why this might have happened. Because the weight at chest level is initially lower than a regular bench press, researchers point out this allows subjects to generate more speed off the chest. Explosive power is gospel in raw bench pressing. If force production subsides, the subjects will not be able to drive through the sticking point as they press up and as each chain link comes off of the ground, more force will be required to complete the lift. Folks are forced to hit the gas! These are Division I baseball players, not elite bench pressers. Since the trial was only nine weeks, I believe even though the subjects in the chain group did not get the specific adaptions from traditional bench presses, they learned how to bench press better because speed is the name of the game, and they were forced to adapt because of the chains.

Basically, it came to the specificity principle or a variable resistance tool that taught specific strategies of explosive bench pressing. Dollars to donuts says a mixed regimen with traditional bench presses and chain bench presses would have reigned superior. Both groups increased strength equally. The principle of specificity was not contradicted; chains for a short time just helped the non-traditional group build more explosive power.

One of the beauties of chains is they can allow people with shoulder issues to keep on pressing. As you lower the barbell to your chest, link by link the chain unloads on the floor. Because of the lighter load in the bottom position, less strain is placed on the shoulder in the vulnerable position on the bottom. This may have also helped the subjects; because of less shoulder pain, they trained harder and more aggressively.

Increased muscle soreness at the end of the nine week trial resulted from increased overload because, generally, as a lifter locks a weight out, force production potential increases. Basically, they don't have to give 100 percent through 100 percent of the movement. Chains are the game changer! The entire range of motion is overloaded, causing a greater Delayed Onset of Muscle Soreness. Chains are a great tool but should not be used 52 weeks out of the year.

Researchers believed this could possibly be explained via eccentric unloading that occurs as the chain links load on the floor one by one. The idea is the eccentric unloading induces an increased/sped up stretch-shorten cycle (SSC) transition and possibly resulting in a within-repetition post activation potentiation (PAP) that permits the lifter to apply faster lifting velocities initially on the upward portion of the bench press, then the goal is to maintain this "head start" out of the gate. Researchers concluded: The use of chains appears warranted when athletes need to lift heavy resistances explosively.

Bar Speed: Barbell Verses Barbell with Chains

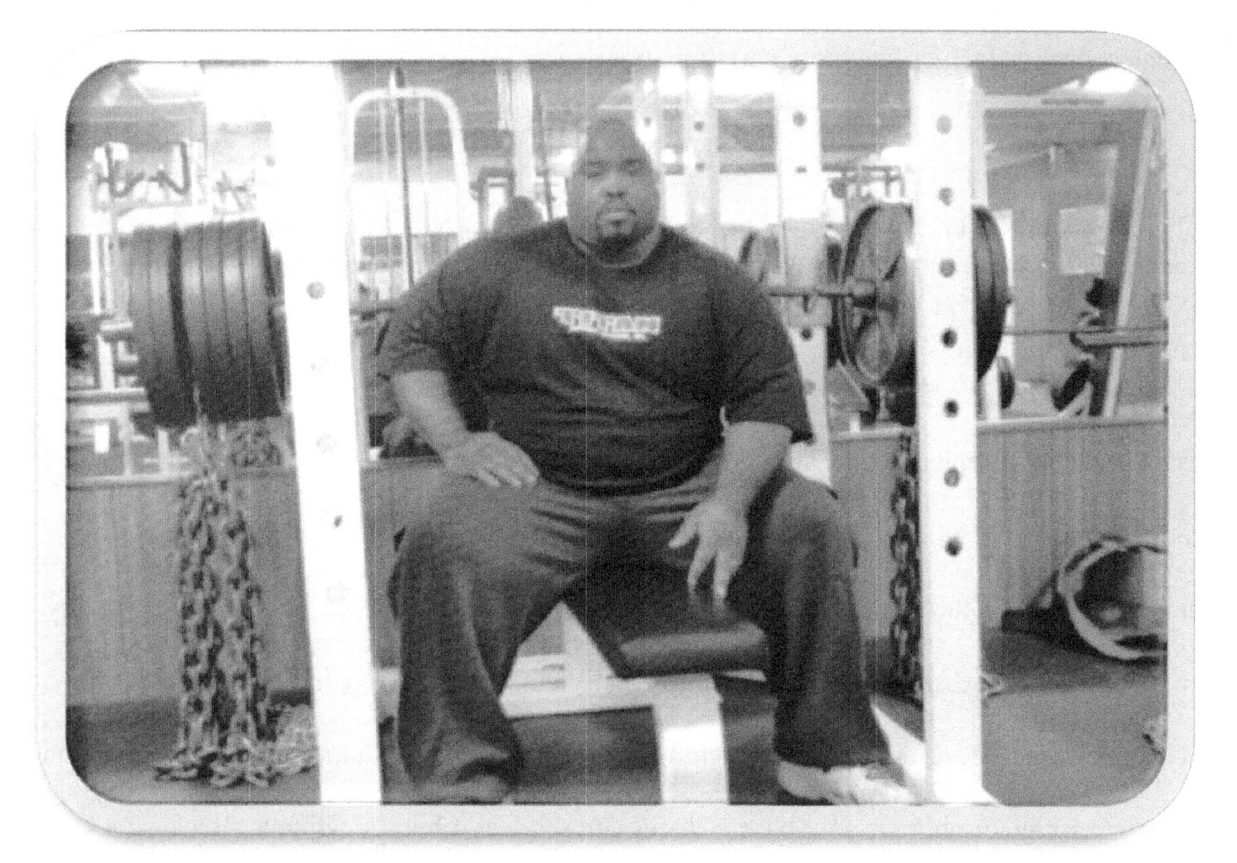

Champion Raw Powerlifter Robert Wilkerson getting ready for heavy bench press with additional chain resistance

The differences in lifting velocity that occur when the bench press exercise is performed with a barbell and weight (traditional) contrasted with a barbell and additional chain resistance were observed. The subjects were 13 professional rugby players with strength training experience. Each athlete bench pressed two sets of three repetitions in the following manner: Bench press barbell+ weights+ chains; the barbell was 60 percent of the athletes' one repetition max (repetition maximum) with an additional 38.5 pounds in chains draped over the barbell (total weight was approximately 75 percent of their one repetition max). The conditions were equal in intensity but with only "straight bar" weight and no additional chains.

The bench press with additional chain weights produced increases in average and maximum concentric lifting velocities of around 10 percent in both sets as compared to straight weight. Eccentric peak velocities had more variation, but in general increased velocity.

Baker, D. G., & Newton, R. U. (2009). Effect of kinetically altering a repetition via the use of chain resistance on velocity during the bench press. *Journal of Strength & Conditioning Research* **(Lippincott Williams & Wilkins), 23(7), 1941-1946.**

Practical Application:

Because chains complement the strength curve of a bench press, they allow the athlete to produce more force longer. Eccentrically, because of the overload, this enhances the elastic energy that will aid the lifter in pushing the weight back up forcefully. Chains physiologically can help increase pressing power and neurologically inhibit potentially inhibitory forces (IE GTO, antagonist effect of biceps). Remember, you have to press in a meet with straight weight, so straight weight training is your base. Chains can serve as a helpful adjunct. Because eccentric muscle actions cause more muscle damage and the chains overload the entire lift, I do not recommend using chains more than three weeks in a row because of potential overtraining.

Final Thoughts

The bulk of your training needs to incorporate the raw bench press with bar weight only. However, bench pressing with bands and chains can serve as a supplement to your bench press training and can help you produce higher amounts of force for longer duration. The choice is not bar weight versus bands and chains; the synergy of using both will help you reap greater results in your raw bench press.

Bench Press: Muscle Activation, Technique, and Volume

Let's take a look at what science has to say.

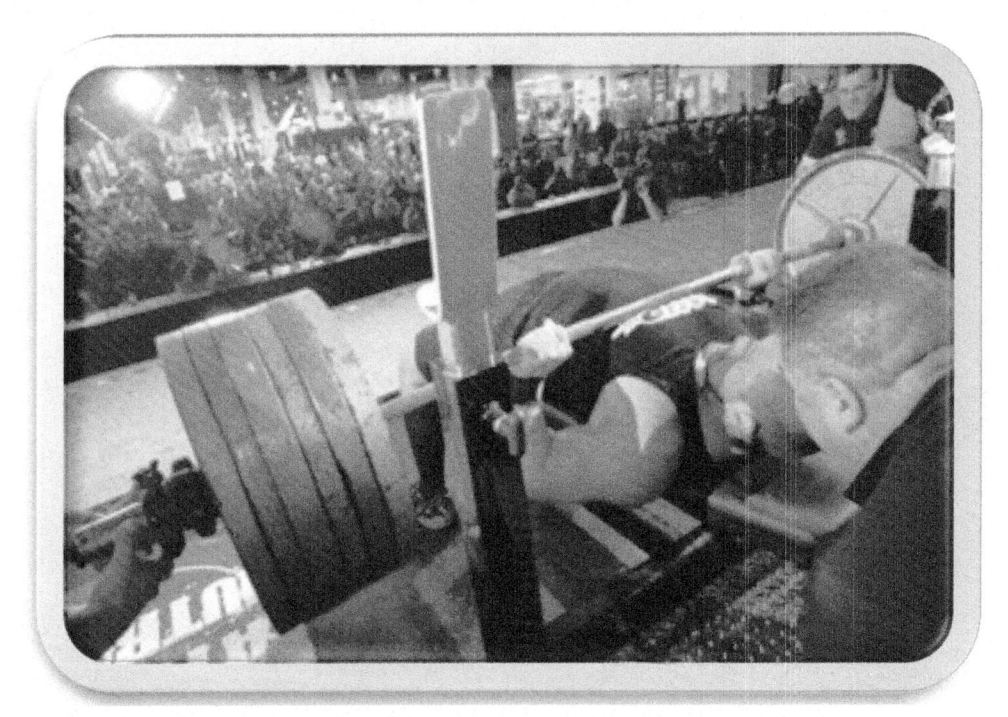

Jeremy Hoornstra in route to breaking his own world record in 2007

Grip Width-Shoulder Safety and Muscle Activation

Most researchers and lifters believe that bench pressing with a narrow grip helps reduce the potential risk of pec tears and shoulder injuries. EMG studies showed that grip width did not cause a major difference in the recruitment of the pecs, but intensified triceps activity.

This study demonstrated that bench press grips wider than shoulder width increased the chance of pec tears and shoulder injuries. Shoulder torque is 1.5 times greater with a wide grip than a narrow grip.

Green, C. M., & Comfort, P. (2007). The Affect of Grip Width on Bench Press Performance and Risk of Injury. *Strength & Conditioning Journal* (Allen Press), 29(5), 10-14.

Practical Application

The wider the grip, the less distance you have to push the bar to complete a bench press. This is why many competitive lifters pick a wide grip for the bench press. Lately, some lifters, including the greatest bench presser of all time, Jeremy Hoornstra, have had success with a narrower grip.

Lifters that espouse narrow grips say this feels better on their shoulders and gives them better drive off the chest.

The whole basis of wide grip bench presses as a supplementary lift is to build drive off the chest. Interestingly, narrow grips had similar chest activation but greater triceps activation. Even though less distance is required to push the barbell with a wide grip bench press, more muscles appear to be activated with a narrow grip. This is certainly something to consider when choosing a grip width because YOU are pushing the weight off your chest, not a bench press shirt. Recreational lifters and athletes should avoid ultra wide grip bench presses. Everything in training has a risk to benefit ratio. Maximum poundages in competition are not the end game! Better safe than sorry by avoiding the wide grip. On the flip side, if world records are the end game, anything totally safe is totally useless.

Factoring in Rest Intervals in Program Design

Rest interval lengths are a common discussion amongst athletes and trainers. This study looked at their effect on bench press performance in subjects across a wide spectrum of bench press abilities. Two cohorts of subjects performed three sets of 10 reps with 75 percent of their one repetition maxes. Rest intervals were 1, 2, or 3 minutes.

The first cohort investigated gender differences in rest intervals studying 22 men and women. The second cohort consisted of 23 men and they were all tested for their one repetition maxes. They were divided into a weak group where maxes ranged approximately 150 to 200 pounds and a strong group where maxes ranged from approximately 280 to 335 pounds.

With one minute rest intervals, women performed significantly more reps than men. The weaker group of men performed more reps than the stronger group. Men's peak power and velocity decreased more than women's during the sets.

The study concluded that maximal strength plays a role in bench press performance with varying rest periods and suggests that shorter rest periods are effective for women.

Ratamess, N. A., Chiarello, C. M., Sacco, A. J., Hoffman, J. R., Faigenbaum, A. D., Ross, R. E., & Kang, J. (2012). The Effects of rest interval length on acute bench press performance: The influence of Gender and muscular strength. *Journal of Strength & Conditioning Research* **(Lippincott Williams & Wilkins), 26(7), 1817-1826.**

Practical Application

I have spent my life in the trenches with clients ranging from socialite women in Santa Barbara, California, to being a strength coach at UCLA, to training some of the strongest men in the world. I have observed that novices need less time to recover than elite lifters, and women less time than men. This is imperative to factor in program design.

It makes perfect sense if you think about it. Advanced lifters activate more motor units because of neural adaptations as they become better lifters. Activating a greater number of high threshold motor units (HTMUs) means greater fatigue. Generally, stronger people have more fast-twitch muscle fibers than weaker folks, and men have more than women. Fast-twitch fibers fatigue faster.

Absolute intensity is the weight on the bar. Relative intensity describes the weight on the bar in relation to your one repetition max. The relationship is not necessarily one to one. This is why rest pause programs are so effective for hard gainers, medium gainers and even faster gainers. The particular effectiveness is amplified for the slow gainer with a rest pause protocol. Because most programs are designed for fast gainers, guys with faster twitch muscle fibers are generally "fast gainers." This means they can do fewer reps with the same relative intensity as a slow gainer; the rest pause program makes it adaptable to the individual.

Since novices and women require shorter rest intervals, plan programs accordingly.

Failure Affects Bar Path

Most bench press training programs utilize multiple repetition sets. There is very little information on how technique (bar path) is affected when taking a set to momentary muscular failure (MMF). This study examined changes in bar path with 18 recreational lifters (10 men and 8 women).

Subjects were tested for a one-repetition max in the bench press. Subjects then performed a maximum number of reps with 75 percent of their one repetition max. Changes in bar path were observed between submaximal and maximal lifts and as subjects approached failure. Obviously, peak power and bar speed decreased as subjects approached failure, and in later repetitions, maximum bar speed was reached earlier in the lift than at commencement of the set. The bar path changed as subjects fatigued, keeping the bar directly over the shoulder during the lift. Bar path between later repetitions and max weights was similar. This study concluded that there are definite changes in bar path for recreational lifters during a set to failure. The authors believe it is extremely important for beginning lifters to train for correct bar path, rather than reaching momentary muscular failure.

Duffey, M. J., & Challis, J. H. (2007). Fatigue effects bar kinematics during the bench press. *Journal of Strength & Conditioning Research* **(Allen Press Publishing Services Inc.), 21(2), 556-560.**

Practical Application

You don't get stronger by missing a lift!

Training to failure is a valuable technique for the advanced bodybuilder in the pursuit of muscle hypertrophy. Powerlifters are after neural adaptations; in other words, becoming more skilled at the lift. Training to failure in the bench press, the lift we are trying to master, can impair neural adaptations. Avoid training the bench press to failure. If you accidently fail once in a while it is not the end of the world. On a chronic basis, it can inhibit your ability to get better at the lift. Maximal lifts have a similar bar path as repetitions with submaximal weight as a lifter fatigues. Some folks in powerlifting have been very anti-reps. Reps teach a lifter to grind reps out. Speed, rate of force development, and the ability to grind are the gateway to big raw bench presses.

The take home point is to learn to grind train some repetitions and avoid training the bench press to momentary muscular failure.

Here is a practical example of a strategy that morphed "Big Al" Davis' ability to grind. The similar rest pausing has taught Vince Dizenzo to grind, too.

Before, a bench press workout for "Big Al" would have looked something like this:

Big Al Davis' Bench Press Workout

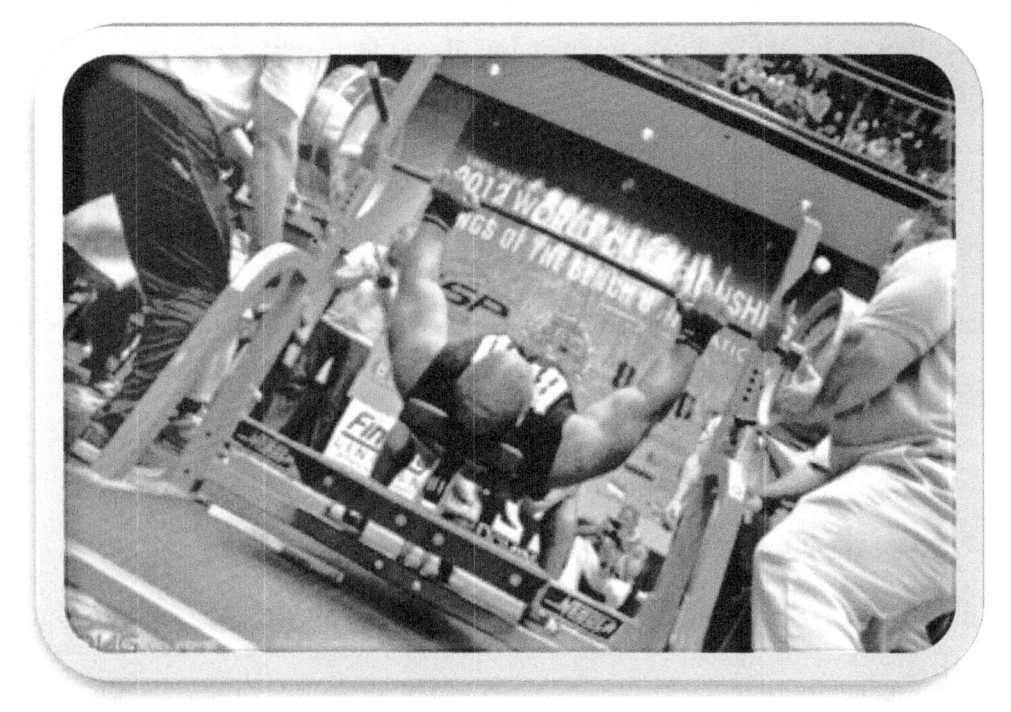

Big Al Davis 500 for reps in Las Vegas

1) Bench Press-645x1 Competition Pause

2) CAT Bench Press-510x3x6 sets (90 seconds break)

With the new strategy purposefully focused on teaching Al to grind, the same workout would become:

Big Al Davis' Rest-Pause Grinding Strength Workout

1) Bench Press-645x1 Competition Pause

2) CAT Bench Press-510x3x6 sets (90 seconds break) (Set 6 would be done in a rest paused style, meaning: Do as many reps as possible stopping one shy of failure, resting 30 seconds, repeating and rest 30 seconds, repeating)

The final CAT set may go something like four reps, two reps, and one rep. Besides teaching Al to grind, this allowed for auto-regulation; meaning, if you feel good, go for it.

Dumbbells, Free Weight, Machines: the Differences

One-repetition maximums and muscle activity in the free weight barbell bench press, smith machine bench press and dumbbell bench press were compared. This study was conducted on 12 healthy, resistance-trained young men.

One-repetition max and electromyographic activity of the pectoralis major, deltoid anterior, biceps, and triceps brachii were documented in the movements. Electrical activity in the pectoralis major and anterior deltoid was similar during all three lifts. As stability requirements increased, electrical activity in the biceps increased. In other words, Smith had the lowest activation of the biceps and dumbbell bench press had the highest activation of the biceps because of having to stabilize the load. Triceps activity was reduced using dumbbells contrasted to barbells.

The study concluded high stability requirements in the dumbbell bench press resulted in similar (pectoralis major and anterior deltoid) lower triceps and higher biceps activation.

Saeterbakken, A. H., Van Den Tillaar, R., & Fimland, M. S. (2011). A comparison of muscle activity and 1-RM strength of three chest-press exercises with different stability requirements. *Journal of Sports Sciences*, 29(5), 533-538.

Practical Application

If stability and staying tight with the weight is an issue, dumbbell bench press provides a scientifically-validated strategy to help attack this weakness. Because biceps play such an important role in stabilizing the weight, it proves curls are not just for girls. Biceps are important muscles in stabilizing heavy weights. A tree with a thick trunk stays stable when the high winds hit, this is not the case with skinny a trunk. This is how biceps work with the bench press. It is rare to see a big bencher with spaghetti arms!

If triceps are a weak point, attack them with a barbell. Triceps activation is lower with dumbbells so band resisted bench press, chain resisted bench presses, board presses and close grips will attack weak triceps and can be complemented with extension variations.

Practice How You Play

It is always exciting to see a study performed on elite lifters. The subjects of this study were Australian male elite bench pressers, with bench press maxes ranging from 330 pounds to 540 pounds.

Bench pressers projected the maximum weight they believed they could max on the bench press the day of the testing. The order of weights bench pressed, following a warm-up, was calculated based on percentages of perceived maximum. The first attempt was 80 percent of perceived maximum, the second was 95 percent of perceived maximum, and the third was the perceived max. A fourth and fifth load of 103 percent and 105 percent were attempted if the lifter was successful with 100 percent.

Each successive attempt from 80 to 105 percent of perceived maximum was only taken if the prior attempt was successful.

Because of prior data analyzed, researchers believed substantial differences occur in both bar path and force profile between a maximal load and a submaximal one. Researchers believed the training effect gained from bench pressing 81 percent of a one repetition max would not offer optimal transference to a maximal load.

Researchers found "Significant differences in bar path and alterations to the general force profile of movement were evident as the load was increased." Because of these alternations, researchers concluded, "(a) The movement pattern adopted during the performance of an 81 percent maximum load was not specific to that which was utilized during the maximal load. (b) Based upon the concepts of specificity of training and testing, the use of the popular one-repetition maximum test to quantify strength changes derived from submaximal training appeared invalid."

Wilson, G. J., Elliott, B. C., & Kerr, G. K. (1989). Bar Path and Force Profile Characteristics for Maximal and Submaximal Loads in the Bench Press. *International Journal of Sport Biomechanics*, **5(4), 390-402.**

Practical Application

As the load in the bench press increases, the movement becomes a different movement. Repetition is the mother skill and the more often we lift a submaximal load with optimal technique, the better bench presser we become. The principle of specificity goes beyond that. To get better at the bench press, you have to bench press, and we have to look at loading parameters. To be the best bench presser you can be, you are going to have to handle heavy weights, loads in the 90-100 percent+ range. As weight increases, technique changes. To lift big, you have to handle big weights!

Bottom line, if you want to be ready for a meet, you have to lift heavy!!!

Technical Differences: Elite and Novice Bench Press

This review provided a technical analysis of bench press performances by powerlifters. Three groups of lifters were evaluated: 9 heavyweight experts, 19 lightweight experts, and 17 light weight novices. Elite light weight and elite heavy weight powerlifters bench pressed with very similar technique. Technique demonstrated by novices was different.

McLaughlin, T. M., & Madsen, N. H. (1984). Bench press techniques of elite heavyweight powerlifters. *National Strength & Conditioning Association Journal*, **6(4), 44.**

Practical Application

Go to any powerlifting meet and watch a beginning bench presser, then watch a seasoned pro. Significant differences exist from how they set up, to how they grip the bar, to lowering the bar and finally pushing the bar back up. Unfortunately, technique is the most under researched component of bench press prowess. Repetition is the mother of skill. Make each repetition count!

How Many Sets?

One and three set training regimens were compared in recreationally trained individuals in the bench press and leg press. Strength gains were greater for the three set group in the leg press and the bench press.

Rhea MR, Alvar BA, Ball SD, Burkett LN (2002). 16(4):525-9. Three sets of weight training superior to 1 set with equal intensity for eliciting strength. *Journal of Strength & Conditioning Research (Allen Press Publishing Services Inc.), 16(4), 525-529.*

Practical Application

Intensity determines gains. To amplify this effect, volume is needed, multiple sets. Counter to what heavy duty training advocates say, it takes more than one set for maximum strength adaptations, regardless of level. Neural adaptations, along with hypertrophy adaptations, are greater with multiple sets. Keep in mind a rest pause set is really multiple sets, not contradicting this finding.

Another Case for Volume

Another study showed greater strength gains in women performing three sets versus a single set. Both groups increased strength significantly in leg extension (multiple-set group, 15 percent;

single-set group, 6 percent). In the bench press, the three set group increased strength by 10 percent, the one set group did not show measurable improvements.

Schlumberger A, Stec J, Schmidtbleicher D (2001). Single- vs. multiple-set strength training in women. *Journal of Strength and Conditioning Research.*15(3):284-9.

Practical Application

Ladies, don't be scared of volume! Studies need to be performed with an even greater number of sets, to find the upper limit on beginners, intermediate and elite lifters. The only place success comes before work is the dictionary; the bench press is no exception.

Final Thoughts

"Bro science" has quite a bit to say about the individual variables that go into proper programming, so does real science; real science needs to be the guiding light.

Science and the Sling Shot

Unfortunately, this does not exist yet! I have a feeling science will validate the Sling Shot shortly. So far, the anecdotes of raw bench press clients suggest this!

When your triceps just wouldn't grow, you decided to declare war on them! The first tour started with skull crushers and ended in defeat...the second tour with pushdowns...now you're on your tenth tour.

"Fixed fortifications are monuments to man's stupidity," to quote General Patton.

It's time to strategize, friends.

The Sling Shot is not just for equipped powerlifters! This contraption is advertised as a supportive mechanism for the upper body that allows you to handle more weight while bench pressing. Believe it or not, it can actually do much more!

The Sling Shot can allow a lifter to handle an additional 10 % of the bench press, so if you can bench 300 pounds, you can now do 330 pounds.

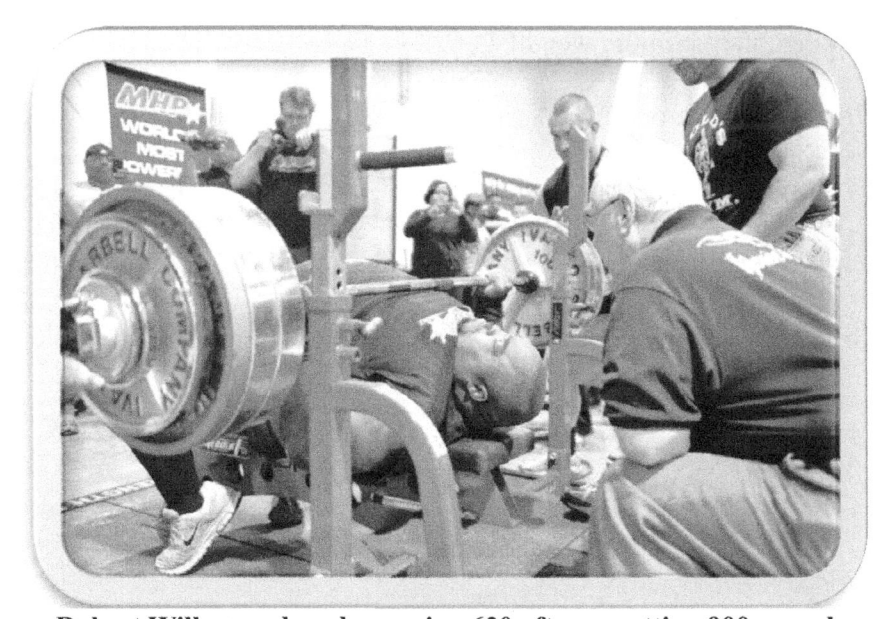

This device is the brain child of Supertraining Gym owner Mark Bell. As an elite lifter, Mark designed the apparatus to mimic natural muscle movement, by lengthening and shortening with the

Robert Wilkerson bench pressing 630 after squatting 900 pounds

muscles. This gives support on the negative and the positive phases of the bench press. Many folks are surprised to learn I have used the sling shot with elite raw bench pressers like Robert Wilkerson and "Big" Al Davis. The reason is simple: you can handle supramaximal weights through a full range of motion. Additionally, stress is reduced on the chest, shoulders and elbows, while overload is placed on the triceps.

A powerlifter or strongman may have a couple months in the off-season to focus attention on strengthening his triceps. Let's say he hits them hard once a week. There is not sufficient time for a gadget like a bench shirt that requires a significant learning curve. You can make the most of your time with a Sling Shot because, unlike a bench press shirt, the Sling Shot is simple to use. Throw it on and go!

Reduced stress on the chest sounds contrary to the fitness fatigue model and development of power off the chest for a full range of motion bench press. The goal is to work your lockout, and handle supramaximal weights, not directly work your chest on the bottom end of the movement. Because of the monstrous loads being used and the reduction of chest and shoulder contribution, the triceps receive a synergistic overload, resulting in you confidently handling larger loads and having better efficiency in locking out maximum weights!

Close grip bench presses with a regular bar or neutral grip bar are a great Sling Shot tricep overload exercise. Weighted dips can be done easily with a Sling Shot. You can handle heavier weights and further increase triceps overload. I have even had a 400-pound general fitness client that did push-ups wearing a Sling Shot, allowing us to work around his shoulder pain and yield satisfactory results.

Here is an example of a powerlifting workout incorporating the Sling Shot:

1) Bench Press-1, 1,3,3,3

2) Close Grip Swiss Bar Press (With Sling Shot)-3x3

3) Front Raises-8, 8, 8

4) Rolling Dumbbell Tricep Extensions-15, 12, 10, 10

5) Reverse Fat Bar Curls-12, 12, 12

Final Thoughts

I have one agenda with this book, to help you increase your raw bench press. Hopefully, we will soon see science reinforce what we have been doing in the trenches for years. To a big Bench Press!

Miscellaneous Bench Press Science

Let's take a look at some other studies that can aid the acquisition of a huge bench press.

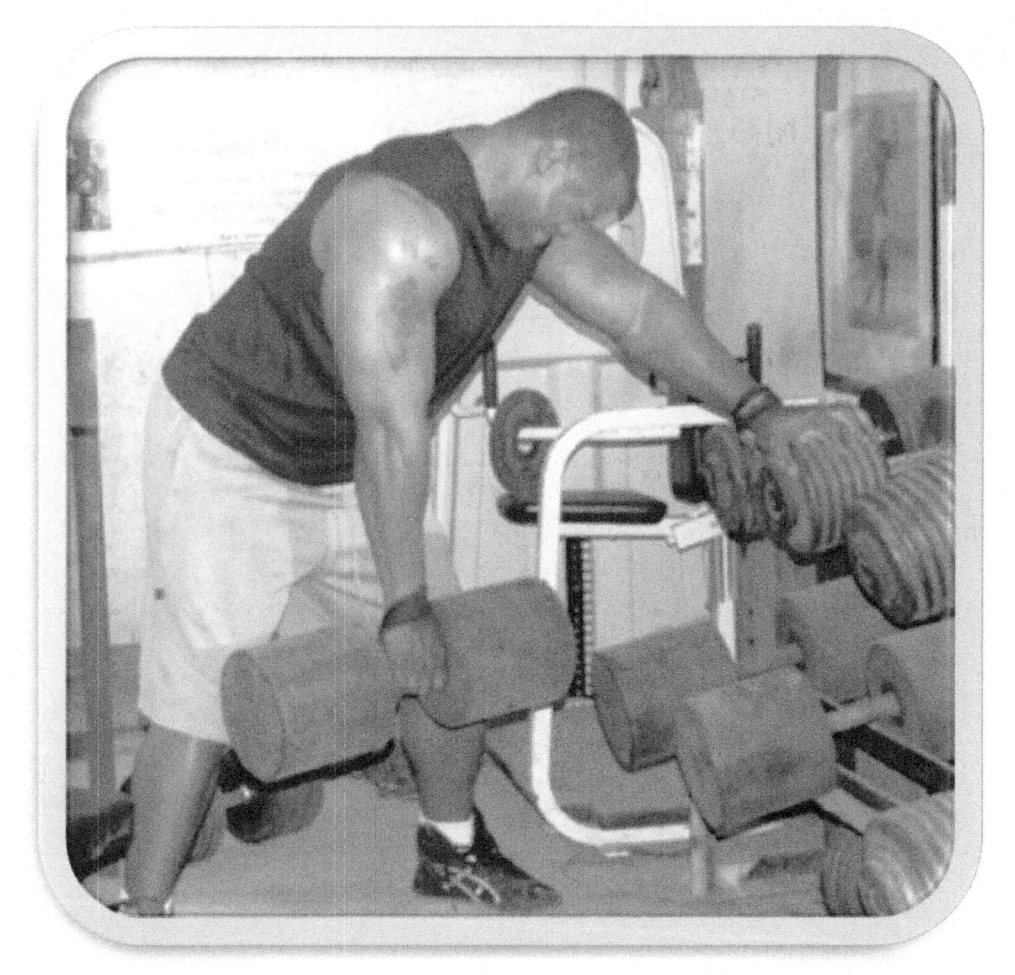

Al Davis heavy dumbbell rows

Curls Are For Girls and So Are Bench Presses

This study had college aged males and females test their one repetition max in the leg press and bench press with a same sex tester present only. Then, they tested on a separate occasion with members of the opposite sex observing their one repetition maxes. Significant increases in both lifts were observed when the opposite sex was present.

J. K.Baker, S.C., Jung, A.P., & Petrella, J.K. (2011). Presence of observers increases one repetition maximum in college-age males and females. *International Journal of Exercise Science*, 4(3), 199-203.

Practical Application

When at the gym, make sure you're concentrating on the task at hand but when maxing out, go ahead and invite your favorite female members to observe.

Take Caffeine and Bench Press More

Abundant studies have shown that caffeine can improve aerobic performance. Does the same hold true with high intensity strength training? This study examined just that and the mechanism of choice was our beloved bench press.

The effect of caffeine was observed (5 mg • kg(-1)) vs. placebo on bench presses to momentary muscular failure (MMF); additionally, subjects' mood post exercise was observed .

Thirteen men with some weight training experience completed two laboratory appointments after their one repetition max in the bench press was determined. Subjects completed bench press repetitions to momentary muscular failure with 60 percent of their one repetition max. Mood was gauged 60 minutes before and instantly post-caffeine ingestion.

Borg's rating of perceived exertion (RPE) and peak blood lactate (PBla) were assessed following each assessment, and peak heart rate (PHR) was figured out. Subjects that consumed caffeine completed significantly more repetitions before reaching failure and had an increased sense of well-being post caffeine consumption.

This study concluded caffeine consumption enhances performance in short-term resistance exercise to failure and can even enhance a positive mind set.

Duncan, M.J. & Oxford, S.W. (2001) The effect of caffeine ingestion on mood state and bench press performance to failure. *Journal of Strength & Conditioning Research* (Lippincott Williams & Wilkins), 25(1), 178-185.

Practical Application:

Caffeine increases the work capacity of muscles and enhances a positive mood. Lift more and feel better by taking a pre-workout with caffeine prior to work out, or drink a strong coffee; a large Starbucks coffee has over 400 mgs of caffeine. The body acclimates to large amounts of caffeine quickly, so I suggest avoiding pre-workout stimulants during deloads and minimizing the consumption of caffeinated beverages.

Pre-workout supplements are not placebos; they are, in fact, backed by science.

Complex Training Saves Time

Complex training means pairing exercises of two opposing muscle groups. In this case, the bench press and the bench pull. Researchers hypothesized that since the bench pull contracts the opposing muscles of the bench press, prime mover muscles of the bench press would be enhanced because the inhibitory effects of the opposing muscles decreases. When you lockout a bench press, the triceps are the prime mover and the biceps oppose it with a built-in safety mechanism to make sure you do not hyperextend your elbow.

Unfortunately, the inhibitorly effect manifests itself far too early, way before true "safety" is actually needed.

Robbins, D. W., Young, W. B., Behm, D. G., & Payne, W. R. (2009). Effects of agonist-antagonist complex resistance training on upper body strength and power development. *Journal of Sports Sciences*, **27(14), 1617-1625.**

Practical Application

Over the course of eight weeks, the complex training group did not have a significant surge in bench press strength over the control group that trained with traditional sets. However, this study demonstrated the efficiency of complex training: the same amount of work could basically be done in half the time without compromising strength gains. Complex training is an effective means of cutting down time in the gym and continually making gains. It is important to note most advanced strength athletes do not train this way. The subjects were not competitive lifters.

Restricting Blood Flow for Strength and Hypertrophy

This study examined the effect of restricting blood flow to the upper arm muscles during a low intensity bench press regimen. Subjects were divided into a control group and a blood flow restricted group. Both groups bench pressed 30 percent of their one repetition max twice daily, six days a week, for four weeks; the workout totaled 75 repetitions.

The blood flow restricted group bench pressed with elastic cuffs on both arms, and pressure increased progressively on both arms, with incremental increases in external compression starting at 100 mmHg and ending at 160 mmHg.

Amazingly, the blood flow restricted group increased muscle thickness in triceps by 8 percent and pectoralis major muscles by 16 percent. Interestingly, the muscle thickness of the control group stayed the same. The control group's one repetition max bench press decreased by 2 percent over the two weeks while the blood flow restricted group's bench press increased 6 percent.

Yasuda, T., Fujita, S., Ogasawara, R., Sato, Y., & Abe, T. (2010). Effects of low-intensity bench press training with restricted arm muscle blood flow on chest muscle hypertrophy: a pilot study. *Clinical Physiology & Functional Imaging*, 30(5), 338-343.

Practical Application

Both groups in this study were novices. Barring injury, no advanced bench presser routinely trains with 30 percent of his one repetition max. Injury is where this study is potentially applicable. When novices start to train, initial strength gains are neural, meaning they get better at the movement; strength gains, because of increased muscle mass, take much longer. By restricting blood flow to the upper arms with light weight, the injured bench presser may be better able to hold on to his bench press limit strength and his hard-earned muscle hypertrophy. This all sounds great on paper. Hopefully, soon a similar study will be performed on healthy elite bench pressers with maximal weights.

Final Thoughts

The goal is a bigger bench press. This information, not falling in a general category, can help you do just that.

Building Bottom End Power

Because speed starts at the bottom, here are a few of my favorite exercises to assist in building bottom end power:

Wide Grip Bench Presses

Physical therapists and corrective exercise gurus have made a strong attempt to hijack the strength game. While many of them offer coaches and strength athletes some great ideas on how to keep things safer, keep in mind that anything that's totally safe is totally useless when it comes to building elite strength. Wide grip bench presses are

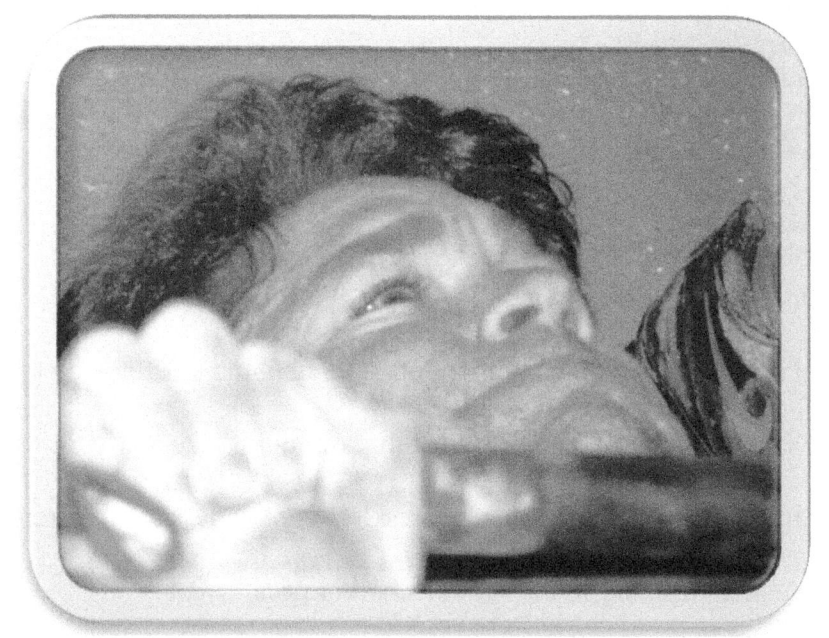

Two-time NCAA shot put champion Noah Bryant getting ready to blast a 500 pound raw bench press into oblivion

very effective for building power out of the bottom of the bench press; a nice byproduct is a muscular chest. Wide grip bench presses were a major reason for my client, Chad Wesley Smith, increasing his bench press max by over 50 pounds in 12 weeks, and they served as a vital part of my arsenal in becoming the youngest person to bench press 600 pounds.

Before I starting working with Jeremy Hoornstra, his world-record raw bench press of was 615 pounds, where it had been for the past five years. Within eight months, he benched an easy 661 raw, arguably the greatest bench press feat of all time. Wide grip bench presses were largely responsible for this massive increase. Any movement that can help the best of the best increase his bench press in epic proportions should make the average lifter take note.

Wide grips were a favorite in building power and speed off the chest of Bill Kazmaier, who bench pressed 661 pounds 30 years ago. Ed Coan religiously used wide grips for years and bench pressed 545 pounds at a body weight of 220 pounds. Powerlifting guru Louis Simmons has advocated wide grips for decades.

The wide grip bench press is performed with a pause. The pause needs to be performed minimally, about as long as a motionless-press command in a powerlifting meet. If you are new to the game, err to the side of a long pause, not a short one; after all, this movement serves to build power off the chest!

This movement was heavily influenced by "illegal wide grips," which means to bench press with a grip wider than the maximal 81 cm allowed in competition. I have found a better way that allows you to handle maximum weights and decrease the probability of injury: take a grip approximately two inches wider than your competition bench press. Do not go less than six reps on this exercise because of the potential of injury to the shoulder and/or pecs.

Perform this exercise in the six to eight rep ranges. A good starting point is 55 percent of your current one repetition paused bench press max. If you pause bench press 200 pounds raw, you will start with 110 pounds for two sets of eight reps. Slowly add weight weekly.

A word of caution: if you have a history of shoulder/pec injuries, avoid this exercise. Everything we do in training is a risk to benefit ratio. The risk will outweigh the benefit if you fall into this category! AVOID THIS MOVEMENT.

Thin lifters with long arms need to generally avoid this movement. Training hard is different than blindly disregarding health.

Cambered Bar Bench Presses

Overload training is associated with heavy partial movements. An alternative overload is increasing the range of motion. Most current top deadlifters perform deficit deadlifts by standing on elevated surfaces to increase their range of motion.

Similarly, this same concept can be applied to the bench press with the cambered bar.

Lifters can increase their range of motion with the cambered bar. The cambered bar has greater stability than dumbbells, meaning more weight can be lifted. Specific transference is greater barbell to barbell.

The cambered bar was the brain child of arguably the greatest bench presser of all-time, Mike MacDonald.

MacDonald bench pressed a world record of 603 pounds in the 242-pound weight class over 30 years ago, a record that stood until 2007. While interviewing Mike for this book, he stated repeatedly that a large part of his success was due to the cambered bar bench press.

Cambered bar bench presses strengthen your chest. MacDonald describes it as, "Hitting the deepest fibers in the chest that are impossible to hit with a straight bar" and went on to say he did this in variety of rep ranges, "doing mostly triples as a meet approached."

Mike MacDonald simultaneously held world records across a spectrum of weight classes and bench pressed 500 lbs raw weekly for at least 15 years consecutively.

A big bench is our objective, so the cambered bar will be used to improve bench press starting strength. Cambered bars have a depth of five inches and Mike and other old school legends performed this full range of motion with it.

Tremendous power was built this way; however, this posed a very high risk of injury. To lessen the risk: shorten the stroke by adding boards to your chest. If you go 1-2 inches past chest level, you are still increasing the range of motion, still building tremendous power off your chest and handling heavier weights while decreasing the chance of injury. Bottom line, too deep is tremendously taxing on the shoulders and pec/delt tie-ins.

The pseudo physical therapist corrective exercise types have dubbed the cambered bar the "shoulder wrecker." This would be a fair assessment if everyone was built the same and had identical genetics. Following the recommended guidelines cuts down the risk of injury but certainly does not eliminate the risk.

Those built to bench: short arms and barrel chested, sans a history of pec or shoulder injuries, should consider this movement.

Conversely, those with long arms who lack a robustly built chest and shoulders and/or have a fair share of injuries should avoid this exercise! Examine the position at the bottom of the bench press, particularly, the angle of your elbow and shoulder joints. Now compare that to someone built to bench. Friend, you are already performing a cambered bar bench press compared to your shorter-limbed, thicker counterparts. Lankier lifters have used this exercise successfully, but for the risk to benefit ratio, it's too far on the risk side.

If you have any history of shoulder or chest issues, regardless of body type, do not perform this movement.

Some key points to remember

- ➢ Increase range of motion by .5 to 2 inches. ROM can be shortened by adding boards to the chest (any more than 2 inches can also alter technique, handicapping transference).

- ➢ Reps should range two to six for strength.

- ➢ Perform a very quick pause at the bottom the movement.

- ➢ Never use bands because of the increased speed of the negative. Chains are okay.

Dumbbell Bench Presses

Like the cambered bar, dumbbell presses can increase the range of motion and can help build power out of the bottom. Dumbbells cause less wear and tear than the cambered bar and allow many with preexisting injuries to reap some of the reward the cambered bar offers. Dumbbell bench presses should be used for 2-4 sets of 6-12 repetitions. No doubt dumbbell bench presses have helped people achieve an immortal status in the bench press. Dumbbells do, however, have some draw backs; it is much easier to cheat with dumbbells. Think of the bodybuilder at the gym that can't bench 300 pounds but does sets of 10 in the dumbbell bench presses with 120s. He is able to do this because he is shortening his range of motion; the heavier you get, the harder it is to tell. This bodybuilder will never know because the squadron of cheerleaders he trains with will never say a peep, and a few people on Facebook liked the video he posted. Let's get back to reality, this is hogwash.

Admittedly, dumbbell bench presses offer less risk than the cambered bar bench press. Dumbbells allow the joints a more free range of motion than the much more fixed access of rotation a barbell forces. Your goal is to increase your barbell bench press. If all else is equal, a better transfer of training will occur with a cambered bar bench press performed with a barbell.

Bottom End Drives

Are you having problems developing starting strength in the bench press? Bottom end drives can be a very helpful adjunct in developing the desired explosive power off the chest. The lift is performed like a normal bench press except instead of driving the bar to full extension from the bottom position, drive the bar half way off the chest, back to the bottom, pause it, and repeat. Do not lock out until the last rep. If you are doing a set of six, you will perform 5 half reps, then lockout the sixth. These are very effective in the 4-6 repetition range. These were a favorite Bill Kazmaier. I learned of these from Kaz in a conversation we shared many years ago at the LA Fitness Expo.

These have been a tremendous asset to building the bench press power of Robert Wilkerson and Jeremy Hoornstra.

Final Thoughts

The bench press has an ascending strength curve; in other words, it is most difficult off the bottom and as leverage improves, so does force production capabilities. It is easier the closer to lockout it gets. The poorest leverage is out of the bottom; the more bottom end power you build, the more you bench press.

Take Home Points

"Experience without theory is blind, but theory without experience is mere intellectual play," said Immanuel Kant.

My goal with this book was not to feed you a fish for a day but to teach you how to fish. You now know the how and the why. The scientifically proven principles presented can serve to help you build a big bench whether you train using conjugate, 5/3/1, The Cube, or anything in between.

Time to get stronger!

Made in the USA
Coppell, TX
04 June 2022